Basic Guide to
Orthodontic Dental Nursing

BASIC GUIDE TO ORTHODONTIC DENTAL NURSING

Second Edition

Fiona Grist

BA (Hons) OU

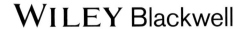

Registered Offices
John Wiley & Sons, Inc., 111 River Street, Hoboken, NJ 07030, USA
John Wiley & Sons Ltd, The Atrium, Southern Gate, Chichester, West Sussex, PO19 8SQ, UK

Editorial Office
9600 Garsington Road, Oxford, OX4 2DQ, UK

For details of our global editorial offices, customer services, and more information about Wiley products visit us at www.wiley.com.

Wiley also publishes its books in a variety of electronic formats and by print-on-demand. Some content that appears in standard print versions of this book may not be available in other formats.

Library of Congress Cataloging-in-Publication Data
Names: Grist, Fiona, author.
Title: Basic guide to orthodontic dental nursing / Fiona Grist.
Other titles: Basic guide to dentistry series.
Description: Second edition. | Hoboken, NJ : Wiley-Blackwell, 2020. |
Series: Basic guide to dentistry series | Includes index.
Identifiers: LCCN 2019035284 (print) | LCCN 2019035285 (ebook) |
ISBN 9781119573692 (paperback) | ISBN 9781119573708 (adobe pdf) |
ISBN 9781119573746 (epub)
Subjects: MESH: Orthodontics | Dental Assistants
Classification: LCC RK521 (print) | LCC RK521 (ebook) | NLM WU 400 |
DDC 617.6/43–dc23
LC record available at https://lccn.loc.gov/2019035284
LC ebook record available at https://lccn.loc.gov/2019035285

Cover Design: Wiley
Cover Image: Courtesy of David Morris

Set in 10/12.5pt Sabon by SPi Global, Pondicherry, India
Printed and bound in Singapore by Markono Print Media Pte Ltd

10 9 8 7 6 5 4 3 2 1

Dedication

For Michael,
with love

Contents

Foreword to Second Edition

The orthodontic team is in the privileged position of being able to significantly improve our patients' lives almost on a daily basis. To do this efficiently and effectively requires not only an understanding of all the equipment and materials available, but precision team-work practised day in, day out.

We, as orthodontists, are totally dependent upon our orthodontic assistants to understand exactly what we are doing and to be able to predict what we are going to require next, to ensure the correct instruments and materials are prepared accordingly. Working with a well-prepared and conscientious assistant is a dream, and ensures high-quality treatment is delivered to as many patients as effectively as possible.

This second edition of the *Basic Guide to Orthodontic Dental Nursing* by Fiona Grist allows the trainee orthodontic nurse to take the first tentative steps on a fascinating and rewarding lifelong journey. It will also provide extremely useful revision for experienced orthodontic assistants of many of the orthodontic concepts we are all required to know intimately.

With its recently updated photographs it now provides an invaluable reference book for all those wishing to learn and improve their orthodontic knowledge.

Professor P.J. Sandler BDS (Hons), MSc, PhD, FDSRCPS, MOrthRCS
President, British Orthodontic Society

How to use this book

The aim of this book is to give the dental nurse in general practice an introduction to the world of orthodontics and orthodontic dental nursing. It may also be helpful to trainee nurses working in an orthodontic environment.

Orthodontics is specialist branch of dentistry and has its own vocabulary. The information in this book is a basic guide, so it does not set out to:

- examine clinical features (why the problem arose)
- cover treatment planning (what is the best choice of treatment)
- treatment mechanics (how the appliances achieve what they do).

Its objective is to describe what the dental nurse needs to know so they can work efficiently at the chairside when treating an orthodontic patient.

If you feel you want to develop your knowledge further there are several excellent orthodontic textbooks available. The career pathways for orthodontic dental nurses are now wide and the possibilities are extensive. Nurses have an important place in the dental team. This book aims to be a helpful first guide on what is hoped be a long and interesting journey.

Different procedures for various treatments are outlined in this book. While it is the nurse's role to assist the clinician, there are areas that are their sole responsibility; these are highlighted in the text in italics.

A quick glance into the stock cupboards and cabinets in an orthodontic surgery reveals quite different contents from that of a general dental surgery. There will be nothing with which to fill teeth or fissure seal, or root canal trays. Anything that helps to irrigate a periodontal pocket, whiten a tooth, prepare abutments for a bridge or fit veneers will be missing. Cupboards in orthodontic units and practices may share the basics, such as mirrors, probes and College tweezers, and use the same alginates and disposable sundries, but beyond that they have very little in common. However, these cupboards are full and it is not possible to cover all materials or equipment that is in use, or every method or procedure.

Just as we had to learn what was needed for restorative, endodontic and prosthetic procedures, we need to learn what is needed for orthodontic treatment, which instruments are used for what procedure and why they are used.

Each chapter will cover a topic, with a short background and guide to what you will need to prepare so that the treatment can be undertaken as efficiently as possible. It is hoped that the photographic examples are helpful, the aim being to show the instruments as clearly as possible. The photographs are not all on the same scale.

This book does not go into detail regarding decontamination and sterilisation. The areas to focus on are those that concern the effect repeated sterilisation has on stiffening box joints on pliers. It can also have a detrimental effect on pliers that have cutting edges. When sterilising pliers and instruments with beaks, always have the beaks open. The same procedures and protocols apply in orthodontics as in other specialties. These you already know. As dental care professionals it is up to the nurse to ensure that they are fully aware and comply with all the current legislation, standards and codes of practice.

As with every skill, be it orthodontic treatment or baking a cake, everyone will have their individual method of working and their favourite tools. There is no hard-and-fast rule that says each procedure must be carried out using only certain instruments in the same way or in an exact order. Every clinician has their preferred methods of working and each and every nurse organises the layout of their trays as they like them. This is as it should be – do what works best for you.

There is a saying,

You don't know what you don't know

This book contains a lot of information but at the same time there will certainly be omissions. Every day brings new materials, new techniques and new treatment philosophies. Orthodontics is inevitably becoming split into specialties within a specialty. The pace of development and change ensures that what is current today is not so tomorrow.

I hope that this book achieves what it sets out to do, which is to provide enough written and visual information for a reasonable grounding of basic knowledge. Its aim is to encourage dental care professionals, especially dental nurses, to understand more about orthodontic nursing.

As trained or trainee dental nurses there is so much that you are already expert at doing, so this book will not cover knowledge you already have or skills you already possess. It does not set out to be comprehensive, but aims to give you a basic insight into the world of orthodontic nursing – it is merely a guide.

Acknowledgements

This is the second time I have written acknowledgements for this book and there are now so many more people to thank! So many that is seems like a mini chapter in itself. Firstly, the tremendous support from my home team: my husband Michael and grand-daughter Kate had unlimited patience when computers, cameras and all manner of technology was out to get me. They just quietly sorted it out. I could not have done it without them.

The format and structure of the original book, which benefited from the expertise and enthusiasm of Alan Hall, has remained, enlarged and hopefully improved. Jo Clark has generously taken over the task as my 'go-to' clinical guru. She has been helpful with providing material for new photographs, advice and encouragement, not least in offering her proofreading skills. Her expert eye looked over my shoulder to ensure I had not got my clinical wires crossed. Also thanks to Maureen Dickinson who tried to make sure I did not leave out major facts whilst busily including the minor ones. They devoted many hours to this and I am truly grateful. Colin Anderson was my 'lay' proofreader, who also spent hours crossing the t's and dotting the i's. My thanks to you all for sharing your expertise so generously and for giving the book the benefit of your time, knowledge and experience with such graciousness.

Special thanks must also go to my young photographer, Kate Meheux, whose contribution to the aesthetic appeal and clarity of this book was huge. She was efficient, knowledgeable and enthusiastic and was a pleasure to work with over the many hours we spent chasing our vision.

I must thank David Morris who again gave permission for the images on the cover, Steven Jones who allowed me to re-use his photographs of TADs, Paul Ward who supplied photographs of fixed lingual appliances, Simon Littlewood who supplied the image of a Barrer spring retainer and Daljit Gill for his RME and cone beam CT images. Tracey Buckfield at NEBDN was helpful with permission to reproduce the Certificate in Orthodontic Nursing Syllabus as was Elena Scherbatykh at the GDC with the Certificate of Orthodontic Therapists Syllabus. The Occlusal Indices are reproduced by kind permission of Professor Steve Richmond and Ortho-Care (UK) Ltd. There were also many images supplied by Alan Hall, and Jo Clark let me photograph a wide variety of her orthodontic goodies. I appreciate the kindness of Alison Williams in sharing her knowledge of aligners with me. My sincere thanks also to Alex Cash, and Wendy Bull in the office, for sending me full records of four of his cleft patients, Douglas, Emily, Georgia and Harvey. I want to thank them specially for kindly agreeing to be part of this book. I have tried to give an idea of their treatment journey and show you how great they look now.

Without a doubt one of the most noticeable aspects of this edition is the updating of many of the clinical photographs. This has been made possible by a generous offer from Jonathan Sandler to access his vast database. I am more than grateful for this and his permission to use these photos in the book and the help given by Sue Mallender and Anne McTighe: merely looking at his seemingly endless files was a masterclass in clinical photography.

Orthodontics has some of the very best supply companies and I appreciate their encouragement and willingness to help. These include Richard Garford, Kelvin Scott and Lisa Howorth at Ortho-Care, David Rees and his helpful staff at TOC, Justyn Gumienna at TB Orthodontics, and Mandy Mills at 3M Unitek. All have been really generous with their time.

I have had the pleasure of working with the Orthodontic National Group for Nurses and Therapists from the beginning. Their contribution to the role of dental nurses today was encouraged by their vision. It would be impossible to include everyone but special mention must go to Janet Robins, Maureen Dickinson, Alex Moss and Sally Dye.

I am grateful to Anjli Patel, Chair of Publications and Joe Noar, Head of Clinical Governance at BOS for their help with permission to use PILs and Guidelines. Anshu Sood and Rod Ferguson kindly allowed me to use the BOS Courses on Impression Taking and Clinical Photography. Ann Wright used all her co-ordinating skills with this too!

My respect for the British Orthodontic Society is unquantifiable. They have long been in the forefront of fostering the 'team' approach in orthodontics in the UK and have blazed a trail for other specialties to follow. The Society has always, and continues to be, hugely supportive of orthodontic nurses and therapists. Thanks to Professor Jonathan Sandler for generously agreeing to write a foreword for this book. Special thanks to Ann Wright, Ann Humphrys and Tony Kearney at BOS headquarters in Bridewell Place for their unflagging good humour and willingness to help and share their expertise. You may not realise it but your bar is high, you really do set the standard.

Caroline Holland first encouraged me to write an article on orthodontic nursing. Initially sure I couldn't, she encouraged me to give it a try, for which I will always be in her debt, as without her I would never have written a word.

Nearly all the names on this page are members of the orthodontic family; they share a passion for their work and have themselves made a significant contribution to their specialty, not to mention their patients, colleagues and the sphere of research. They have been gracious in sharing their expertise. All omissions and errors are down to me.

Huge thanks to the team at Wiley-Blackwell, especially Loan Nguyen, Susan Engelken, Jayadivya Saiprasod, Jolyon Phillips, Baskar Anandraj and Nick Morgan. Knowing you were there was good, but hearing your voices at the end of the phone was better. Thanks for all the hand holding.

Last, but by no means least, to you, who have made it to the bottom of the page. Teachers of English will say this piece is woeful as it repeats the words 'generous', 'thanks' and 'appreciate' too often. They are correct but these words are precisely what this page is all about. I hope that you feel inspired to keep turning the pages and that you begin, or are continuing, to enjoy your work in orthodontics, probably the best job in the world!

Chapter 1

Definition of orthodontics and factors influencing orthodontic treatment

Orthodontics is a specialised branch of dentistry. The name comes from two Greek words:

- *orthos*, meaning straight or proper
- *odons*, meaning teeth.

So the meaning is clear – 'straight teeth'.

Orthodontics is the study of the variations that occur in the development and growth of the structures of the face, jaws and teeth and of how they affect the occlusion of the teeth. Ideally there should be the same number of permanent teeth in each arch.

Any deviation from the norm that affects teeth alignment and the bite relationship is called a malocclusion. Most malocclusions are genetic – they are inherited (e.g. missing teeth or a protruding mandible). Other malocclusions can be caused by the patient, for example digit sucking, or by external factors such as trauma.

Orthodontic treatment can correct a malocclusion by restoring the teeth to their normal position and occlusal relationship (with surgical help if needed) so that:

- the bite is fully functioning and the patient can bite and chew properly
- oral hygiene is made easier, so helping to prevent caries and gingivitis
- the malocclusion does not cause other damage, often to soft tissues
- the patient looks better and has better self-esteem.

Orthodontic treatment in conjunction with orthognathic (maxillofacial) surgery can correct an underlying jaw discrepancy or facial asymmetry. Orthodontic planning is done in conjunction with the surgeons using clinical and radiographic assessment, with a cephalometric tracing (Figure 1.1) often analysed using a computer software program.

So orthodontists set out to:

- straighten teeth
- improve the bite
- improve the function
- improve oral hygiene (making teeth easier to clean)
- improve self-esteem of the patient.

Basic Guide to Orthodontic Dental Nursing, Second Edition. Fiona Grist.
© 2020 John Wiley & Sons Ltd. Published 2020 by John Wiley & Sons Ltd.

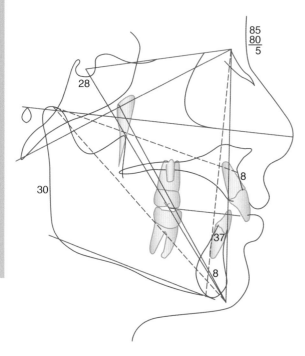

Figure 1.1 Cephalometric tracing.
Source: Reproduced by kind permission of
Alan Hall.

CLASSIFICATION OF OCCLUSION

When assessing occlusion there are two aspects to classification:

- incisor relationship
- buccal segment occlusion, left and right.

Both are recorded on a patient's orthodontic assessment form.

Incisor classification

- classes have Roman numerals, e.g. I, II, III.
- divisions do not, e.g. Class II/1 or Class II/2.

    The incisor classification (Figure 1.2):

- relates to the bite of the tip of the lower central incisors onto the back of the upper central incisors
- it is divided into three horizontal sections and where the lower incisor occludes will determine the classification.

Class I
- the incisal edge of the lower incisors bite on or below the cingulum plateau of the upper incisors.

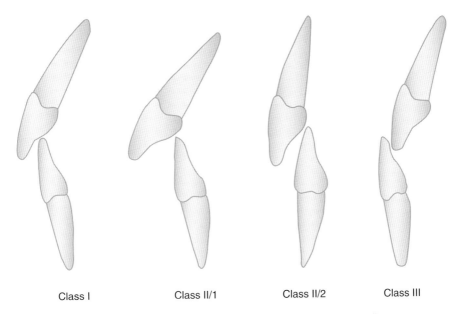

Class I   Class II/1   Class II/2   Class III

Figure 1.2 Incisor classification. Source: Reproduced by kind permission of Alan Hall.

Class II/1
- the upper incisors are proclined or upright (Figures 1.3 and 1.4).
- the lower incisors bite behind the cingulum plateau of the upper incisors.
- the position of these front teeth means they can be damaged more easily because of their vulnerable position.

Class II/2
- the upper incisors are retroclined.
- the lower incisors bite behind the cingulum plateau.
- the position of the teeth can, when closed, lead to trauma to the lower labial gingivae and the upper palatal gingivae (Figures 1.5–1.7).

Class III
- the bite is edge to edge or reversed.
- the incisal edge of the upper incisors can bite into the back (lingual) surface of the lower incisor (Figure 1.8).
- a horizontal overlap is called an **overjet**.
- a vertical overlap is called an **overbite**.

Buccal segment occlusion

The buccal segment occlusion:

- was devised by Edward Angle in 1890
- is still widely used today

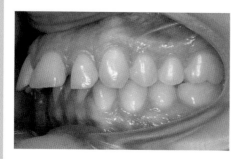

Figure 1.3 Large overjet. Source: Reproduced by kind permission of Jonathan Sandler.

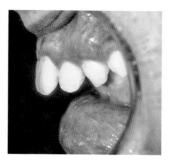

Figure 1.4 Side view of severe overjet. Source: Reproduced by kind permission of Alan Hall.

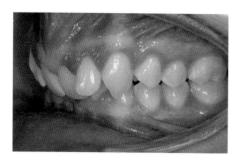

Figure 1.5 Bite stripping lower gingivae. Source: Reproduced by kind permission of Jonathan Sandler.

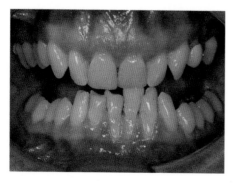

Figure 1.6 Damage to labial gingivae caused by the bite. Source: Reproduced by kind permission of Jonathan Sandler.

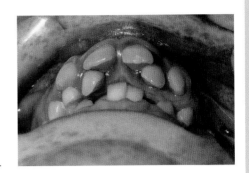

Figure 1.7 Bite causing trauma to the palate. Source: Reproduced by kind permission of Alan Hall.

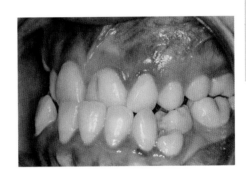

Figure 1.8 Class III. Source: Reproduced by kind permission of Alan Hall.

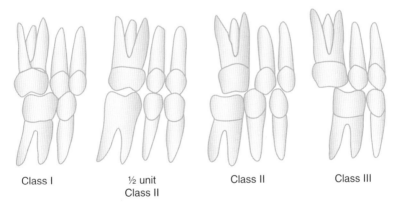

| Class I | ½ unit
Class II | Class II | Class III |

Figure 1.9 Diagram of buccal segment occlusion. Source: Reproduced by kind permission of Alan Hall.

- is based on the occlusion between the first permanent molar teeth, which erupt when the patient is about 6 years old.

  There are three classes:

- **class I:** this is near to the correct relationship
- **class II:** this is at least half a cusp width behind the ideal relationship
- **class III:** this is at least half a cusp width in front of the ideal relationship (Figure 1.9).

THE MIXED DENTITION

Sometimes parents see their child's perfectly straight deciduous teeth fall out only to be replaced by a 'jumble' of crowded permanent teeth. This often prompts them to want early treatment because permanent teeth can look huge in little faces.

Hypodontia

Patients with hypodontia do not have the full complement of teeth. This can occur in the deciduous and permanent dentition. In some cases, if it is just a single tooth, it is possible to close the space orthodontically. If there are too many missing this may require a solution involving replacements such as bridges and implants, with orthodontic treatment being used to position the teeth in the correct spaces (Figure 1.10).

The average times for permanent tooth eruption are as follows.

- age 6
  - 1/1 lower central incisors
  - 6/6 lower first molars
  - 6/6 upper first molars
- age 7
  - 1/1 upper central incisors
  - 2/2 lower lateral incisors
- age 8
  - 2/2 upper lateral incisors
- age 11
  - 3/3 lower canines (cuspids)
  - 4/4 lower first premolars (bicuspids)
  - 4/4 upper first premolars (bicuspids)
- age 12
  - 3/3 upper canines (cuspids)
  - 5/5 lower second premolars (bicuspids)
  - 5/5 upper second premolars (bicuspids)
  - 7/7 upper second molars
  - 7/7 lower second molars

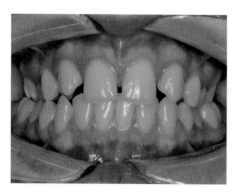

Figure 1.10 Hypodontia. Source: Reproduced by kind permission of Jonathan Sandler.

- age 18–25
  - 8/8 upper third molars (wisdom teeth)
  - 8/8 lower third molars (wisdom teeth).

Normally, patients begin orthodontic treatment between the ages of 10 and 13 years old. At 10–11 years they are still in the mixed dentition, with

- some deciduous teeth
- some permanent teeth
- some teeth yet to erupt.

INDICATIONS FOR TREATMENT

Clinical indications for orthodontic treatment may be because the teeth:

- are overcrowded
- may have erupted out of position
- are protruding (Class II/l)
- exhibit reverse bite
- exhibit self-damaging bite (Figure 1.11)
- are spaced
- are absent (hypodontia)
- are damaged.

Mild malocclusions, for example:

- with only very small irregularities
- where the tooth position does not compromise oral hygiene
- which do not interfere with function, such as biting off food and eating,

may not be merit orthodontic treatment, as it may not be seen to significantly improve dental health.

However, some presentations, for example:

- with overcrowded, protruding teeth
- with rotated teeth that make oral hygiene difficult and cause problems with caries
- which visually deviate from average, e.g. a reverse bite

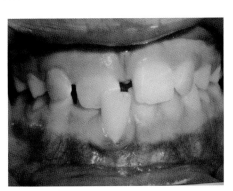

Figure 1.11 Lower incisor trapped outside the bite.
Source: Reproduced by kind permission of Alan Hall.

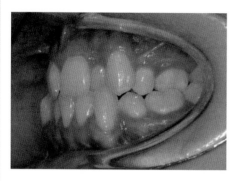

Figure 1.12 Scissors bite. Source: Reproduced by kind permission of Jonathan Sandler.

- which look unattractive and affect the smile
- which seriously affect function, e.g. make chewing food difficult,

are classed as malocclusions warranting treatment.

Scissors bite

This is a lingual crossbite, where the buccal cusps of the lower premolars and molars occlude palatal to their opposing upper tooth (Figure 1.12).

UNDERLYING CAUSES OF MALOCCLUSION OF THE TEETH

There may also be:

- underlying skeletal abnormalities
- facial asymmetries.

These can be:

- hereditary (e.g. tendency to being Class III)
- a result of injury
- a result of illness affecting facial or skeletal growth
- a result of a syndrome or cleft.

These may require orthodontic treatment as part of a multidisciplinary care treatment pathway.

Multidisciplinary approach

In cases requiring a multidisciplinary approach, patients receive their orthodontic treatment in co-ordination with other specialties.

These specialties include:

- restorative (e.g. hypodontia patients requiring implants/bridges or microdontia patients needing veneers or crowns)
- surgical (e.g. patients needing an osteotomy)
- cleft (e.g. patients requiring alveolar bone grafting).

PROBLEMS WHEN THE ARCH IS NOT INTACT

One of the aims of orthodontic treatment is to have each tooth in its correct place within the dental arch.

If a tooth is malaligned (out of its correct position), it is not necessarily an isolated problem – it has a 'domino' effect. The teeth either side of it may also be out of their correct position and the opposing tooth does not have the correct occlusion.

If there is no tooth to oppose it, a tooth may supra-erupt. Contact points are lost, teeth rotate and, because they are no longer self-cleansing, food traps are created where fibres can get lodged or packed. As a consequence of this, plaque is encouraged to accumulate, which in turn:

- inflames the gingivae
- encourages periodontal pockets.

In the young patient this is not too drastic, as it probably has not yet become a significant issue.

In adult patients, however, following orthodontic treatment it may be necessary to restore incisal edges or fill cervical abrasion cavities, which only become apparent when the teeth have been corrected.

BRUXISM

- young patients, towards the end of the deciduous dentition, can often present with teeth almost ground down to gingival level. It may continue into the mixed dentition and is often quite noisy and noticeable when it occurs in sleep.
- for some older patients with severe bruxism, an occlusal guard can be made to be worn at night during sleep. This attempts to limit the damage that is done to the incisal and occlusal surfaces of the teeth.
- anxious patients also grind and clench their teeth during the day when under stress. Patients often also clench their teeth when doing weight training at the gym.

DIGIT SUCKING

Some patients continue to suck their fingers or thumbs well beyond the age when their deciduous teeth have been replaced by their permanent successors. A prolonged habit is one which exists until the age of 7 years.

It may adversely affect the bite and position of the anterior teeth and can produce:

- a unilateral buccal crossbite
- an asymmetrical anterior open bite where the finger or thumb enters the mouth (Figure 1.13)
- an increased overjet.

DEFINITION OF ORTHODONTICS

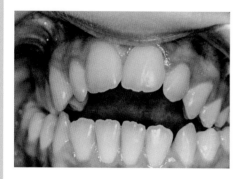

Figure 1.13 Anterior open bite due to digit sucking. Source: Reproduced by kind permission of Alan Hall.

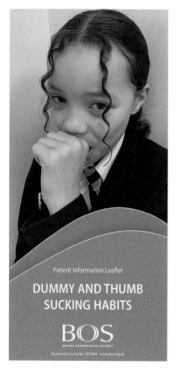

Patient Information Leaflet

DUMMY AND THUMB SUCKING HABITS

BOS
BRITISH ORTHODONTIC SOCIETY
Registered Charity No 1073464 www.bos.org.uk

Figure 1.14 Leaflet on digit sucking. Source: Reproduced by kind permission of British Orthodontic Society.

How much damage is caused depends on how long, and how frequently, the thumb or finger is sucked and how strong the habit is (i.e. occurs not just when alone going to sleep but also during the day when tired, bored or stressed).

These patients try really hard to break this habit but sometimes they need a bit of help (Figure 1.14). It is possible to fit a removable upper anti-habit appliance, which has prongs in the centre of the palate that act as a positive deterrent for the thumb or finger. This is worn full time or only when the individual is asleep.

Once the habit is broken, the problem is often solved. However, some patients experience strong emotional comfort from digit sucking and this compulsion may need to be assessed in detail. An image of an anti-habit device is provided in Chapter 7.

DENTAL HEALTH

Some problems are caused by:

- diet (too much sugary or acidic food or drink, causing dental caries)
- tooth brushing (the wrong technique, too hard a brush)
- acid reflux (a symptom of bulimia in anorexic patients)
- medication (side effect of some medication inhalers).

Damage to teeth resulting in tooth surface loss comes under the following general headings:

- attrition: bruxism (patients who grind their teeth, often during sleep)
- abrasion: excessive wear (e.g. overenthusiastic tooth brushing)
- erosion: of the enamel by acid, found in fresh fruit juice, diet drinks and stomach acid (found in reflux)
- abfraction: a tooth being 'high on the bite' and being overloaded.

Charting of teeth is an area you all know well, and follows the standard numbering commonly used in the UK.

Permanent dentition (as the clinician looks at the patient)

Upper right	upper left
87654321	12345678
Lower right	lower left
87654321	12345678

Deciduous dentition (as the clinician looks at the patient)

edcba	abcde
edcba	abcde

There are other methods of tooth numbering, of which the World Dental Federation (FDI) and the universal numbering systems, are notable examples. Sometimes you may receive transfer cases which use an alternative method to the one you are used to, so it is good to know the alternatives.

The FDI code is one most commonly used and it uses the existing numbers but just adds an extra number:

- upper right is 1, so upper right canine would be 13
- upper left is 2, so upper left lateral would be 22

- lower left is 3, so lower left wisdom tooth would be 38
- lower right is 4, so lower right first premolar would be 44.

And in the deciduous dentition

- upper right is 5, so upper right lateral is 52
- upper left is 6, so upper left canine is 63
- lower left is 7, so lower left central 71
- lower right is 8, so first lower right molar is 84.

CONDITION OF THE SURROUNDING SOFT TISSUES

Lips

- competent: when they are at rest and come together easily and form a good oral seal.
- incompetent: when at rest do not close, or if they are closed, the lips are strained, often as a result of posturing. This closure is only temporary.

Tongue

- the tongue works with the lower lip to form a seal when swallowing.
- a tongue which tends to thrust can push forward and 'splay' the front teeth out.

The position of the teeth and the form of the dental arches are determined by the balance of the soft tissues between tongue and lips/cheek. If the tongue's free movement is restricted, when the lingual frenum is attached too far forward on the tongue, this interferes with, and restricts, function and is called a tongue tie. It can also interfere with speech, hence the expression 'to be tongue tied' (Figure 1.15).

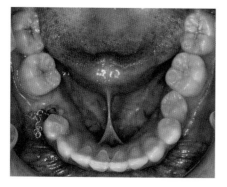

Figure 1.15 Tongue tie. Source: Reproduced by kind permission of Jonathan Sandler.

Chapter 2

The first appointment

Orthodontic patients are usually referred by their own dentist (their general dental practitioner) for specialist orthodontic treatment.

These referrals can be sent to:

- an orthodontic specialist practitioner
- a community orthodontist
- a consultant orthodontist
- a GDP with enhanced skills.

Some adult patients may choose to self-refer.

The referring dentist may wish to send the patient to an orthodontist to:

- see and advise
  - if there are teeth that are slow to erupt
  - if there are teeth that have submerged
  - if there are teeth in a self-damaging position
- see and monitor
  - if the patient is dentally too young for treatment
  - if there are already signs of adverse dental development, i.e. growth, facial asymmetry or crowding
- see and treat
  - if the second dentition has developed but is overcrowded
  - if there is a complex problem
  - if there is a multidisciplinary need.

The referral letter needs to contain as much relevant information for the orthodontic practitioner as possible.

Apart from basic personal data, such as:

- name
- address
- telephone numbers (land, mobile, work, etc.)
- date of birth
- National Health number (if relevant)

Basic Guide to Orthodontic Dental Nursing, Second Edition. Fiona Grist.
© 2020 John Wiley & Sons Ltd. Published 2020 by John Wiley & Sons Ltd.

- name of GP (doctor)
- name of GDP (dentist),.

it also needs to give:

- clinical reason for referral (what the dentist feels is the problem)
- medical history (if it is helpful to know in advance, e.g. attention deficit hyperactivity disorder, autism, deafness, dental phobia)
- dental history (good oral hygiene, high caries level, etc.)
- any previous orthodontic history (e.g. previous assessment or treatment)
- social history (e.g. supportive family, regular check-ups)
- what concerns the patient/parent ('fangs', teasing)
- whether the patient is bothered at all (quite happy to stay as they are)
- likely compliance (supportive family, the patient is keen).

When the referral letter is received, the patient (or their parent or guardian if they are under age) is sent an appointment.

On the first visit a full orthodontic assessment is carried out (Figures 2.1 and 2.2). This includes:

- checking the name and age of the patient
- what is of concern to the patient
- full medical history, including whether the patient
  - has any known allergies (nickel, latex, etc.)
  - is currently under the care of a doctor for any reason
  - has had any operations
  - is taking medication of any kind
  - has asthma; if so, which type of inhalers
  - has diabetes
  - has or had chest or heart conditions.

Patients and/or parents are also asked to fill in and sign a health questionnaire. This should be updated and checked regularly.

This also contains details of:

- school or college (day or boarding)
- work
- contact sports
- musical instruments played by mouth
- any digit (thumb or finger) sucking, bruxism (tooth clenching or grinding)
- lip, cheek or tongue jewellery, e.g. studs
- any known allergies, e.g. latex, nickel.

THE CLINICAL ASSESSMENT RECORDS

These begin with extra-oral features and then move on to intra-oral ones.

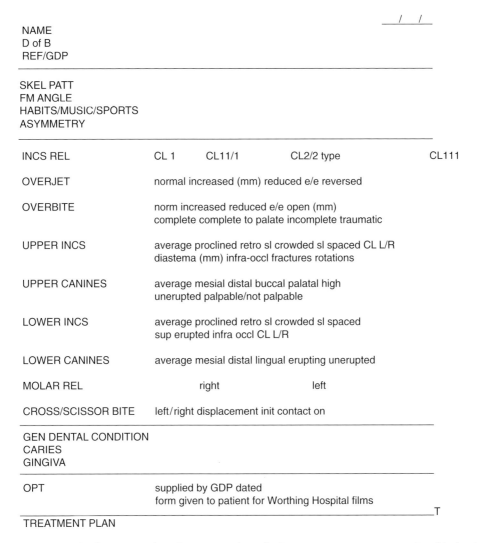

THE FIRST APPOINTMENT

Figure 2.1 Sample of assessment form from a specialist orthodontic practice. Source: Reproduced by kind permission of Alan Hall.

Skeletal pattern

The maxilla to mandible relationship in the antero-posterior plane:

- class I
- class II
- class III
  - mild
  - moderate
  - severe.

THE FIRST APPOINTMENT

ORTHODONTIC CONSULTATION -

Patient Details Age: years months	Medical History	Dental History

Complaint	Social Details

Skeletal Pattern

AP 1 2 3	Vertical ↑ ↓ Average	Lateral Asymmetry Yes No

Soft Tissue Pattern

Lips Competent Incompetent	Lip Line High Low Average	Habit Yes No

Teeth Present ———┼———	**Missing Teeth** ———┼———

Tooth Quality	**Oral Hygiene**	**Caries/Decalcification**
Good Fair Poor	Good Fair Poor	———┼———

Lower Labial Segment

	Mild Mod Severe	*Mild Mod Severe*		
Aligned	Crowded	Spaced	Proclined Retroclined Average	CL L R Centre

Upper Labial Segment

	Mild Mod Severe	*Mild Mod Severe*		
Aligned	Crowded	Spaced	Proclined Retroclined Average	CL L R Centre

Lower Buccal Segments	Aligned Crowded Spaced

Upper Buccal Segments	Aligned Crowded Spaced

In Occlusion	OJ ↑ ↓ Average mm
	OB ↑ ↓ Average Complete Incomplete

Molar Relationship Right	I II III $\frac{1}{4}$ $\frac{1}{2}$ $\frac{3}{4}$ 1
Molar Relationship Left	I II III $\frac{1}{4}$ $\frac{1}{2}$ $\frac{3}{4}$ 1

Incisor Relationship	I II/i II/ii III

Crossbites Yes No	———┼——— Displacement Yes No

Figure 2.2 Sample of assessment form from a hospital orthodontic department. Source: Reproduced by kind permission of Jo Clark.

FM (Frankfort–mandibular) angle (Figure 2.3)

- high
- average
- low.

Asymmetry

- this is usually mandibular.

Soft tissues

Lips
- line (if high, is there a 'gummy' smile)
- competency (do they close when resting)
- expressive behaviour
- if lower lip is behind upper incisors.
  (This is the end of the extra-oral examination.)

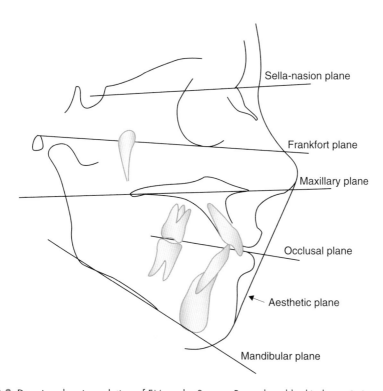

Figure 2.3 Drawing showing relation of FM angle. Source: Reproduced by kind permission of Alan Hall.

Tongue
- size
- position in mouth
- swallowing behaviour
- presence of a tongue tie.

Tonsils
- if there is a history of difficulties in breathing through the nose, snoring or repeated sore throats.

Frenum
- upper
- lower.

Gingivae and oral hygiene

- health of the gums
- presence of plaque.

Charting of the teeth

- present
- absent (unerupted or extracted)
- presence of caries/restorations/fissure sealant
- erosion
- enamel hypomineralisation
- hypoplasia
- size discrepancy:
  - microdont, small tooth (microdontia)
  - megadont, large tooth (megadontia)
- supernumeraries, i.e. teeth which are additional to the norm:
  - most often found in the anterior maxilla
  - can be conical, supplemental or tuberculate.

Incisor relationship (Figure 2.4)

- class I
- class II/1
- class II/2
- class III.

Overjet

Horizontal measurement between upper and lower incisors:

- normal (3 mm)
- increased (record the measurement in millimetres)
- edge to edge
- reversed.

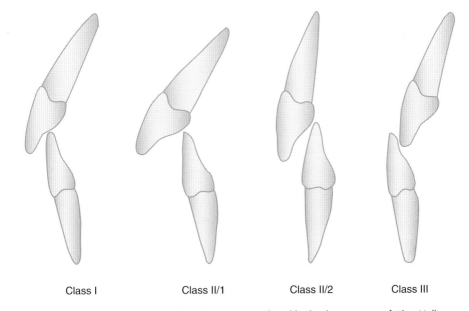

| Class I | Class II/1 | Class II/2 | Class III |

Figure 2.4 Diagram of incisor relationship. Source: Reproduced by kind permission of Alan Hall.

Overbite

Upper incisors overlapping lowers in vertical plane:

- normal
- increased
- reduced
- edge to edge
- open (record the measurement in millimetres)
- complete
- complete to palate
- incomplete
- traumatic.

Upper and lower incisors

- average inclination
- proclined
- retroclined
- crowded
- rotations
- spaced
- diastema (record space in millimetres)
- centreline

- infra-occluded
- supra-erupted
- any fractures/restorations
- any abnormal mobility
- mesial or distal
- buccal or palatal.

Upper canines

- average inclination
- high
- unerupted but palpable
- unerupted but not palpable
- mesial or distal
- buccal or palatal.

Lower canines

- average inclination
- mesial
- distal
- buccal
- lingual
- erupting
- unerupted.

Molar relationship (buccal segment occlusion) (Figure 2.5)

- class I
- ½ unit class II
- class II
- class III.

Crossbite

- localised
- unilateral (arch widths do not match one side)
- bilateral (arch widths do not match both sides).

Scissors bite

- lingual crossbite of lower teeth.

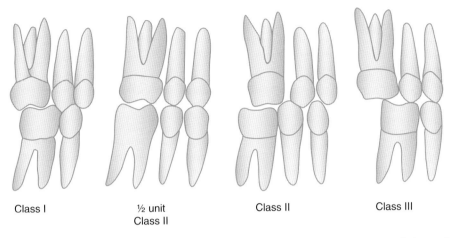

Class I   ½ unit   Class II   Class III
                 Class II

Figure 2.5 Diagram of buccal segment occlusion. Source: Reproduced by kind permission of Alan Hall.

Open bite

* anterior
* posterior
* lateral.

Displacement of mandible when closing

* left
* right
* anterior
* initial contacts.

NB This distinguishes the term from displacement of teeth in the Index of Orthodontic Treatment Need (IOTN).

Note must also be made of:

* submergence (teeth that have 'sunk' down back into the gum)
* impactions
* damaged teeth (e.g. repaired/unrepaired, root filled or ankylosed)
* teeth with a poor-quality long-term outlook (e.g. heavily filled or hypoplastic)
* any transpositions (teeth in exchanged positions, e.g. a canine mesial to a lateral)
* any other anomalies.

There is a 'benchmark' to achieving the ideal occlusion known as the six Andrews' keys, comprising:

* class I molars
* correct incisor inclination
* correct tip
* no spaces

- no rotations
- flat curve of Spee.

It is important at this stage to discuss with the patient exactly what they feel is wrong and what they are hoping to achieve. Sometimes a patient comes in with a very obvious orthodontic problem which would seem to members of the clinical team to be their main concern. However, this may not be the case. Their worry can be a relatively mild problem but to the patient this may be what they want to have changed.

It may also be that what the patient is asking is just not feasible and if this is the case the patient must be advised accordingly. In order to give informed Consent the patient and/or their parent or guardian must fully appreciate the advantages and disadvantages of treatment, all the options possible, and even that the problem cannot be resolved to the extent to which they hoped.

RADIOGRAPHS

If the orthodontist wants to further assess the patient, then radiographs are needed. These are an invaluable diagnostic tool when formulating a treatment plan.

The two formats most routinely used in orthodontic assessment are the orthopantomogram (OPT) and the lateral cephalometric radiograph.

The orthopantomogram (Figure 2.6)

This is an extra-oral radiograph that:

- is a panoramic view of both the maxilla and mandible
- shows all the underlying skeletal structures, including:
  - temporo-mandibular joints (TMJs)
  - position of the condyles (head of the rami)
  - level of alveolar bone (in older patients there can be bone loss)
  - sinuses
  - position of dental nerve canals (e.g. inferior dental nerve)
  - any cysts
  - radiolucencies.
- also shows the dental features:
  - position of the teeth
  - any unerupted or impacted teeth

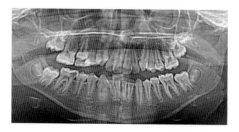

Figure 2.6 Example of OPT radiograph. Source: Reproduced by kind permission of Jonathan Sandler.

- any ectopic teeth (teeth that have developed and erupted or not erupted in their correct position)
- supernumerary teeth
- any anomalies of the teeth (e.g. fusing of roots)
- presence of third molars
- indicate the condition of any teeth that may have cavities or deep restorations (these may influence any decision on the possible need for extractions).

NB OPTs are not taken to show caries but often do. Bite-wing radiographs are needed if there is concern regarding cavities.

The lateral cephalometric radiograph (Figure 2.7) is an extra oral radiograph that:

- shows a true lateral image of the skull and face
- shows angulation of incisor teeth
- is used to monitor skeletal growth, e.g. if the mandible is developing adverse forward growth (Class III)
- may be used to carry out cephalometric tracings for surgical planning in cases with severe skeletal disproportion.

Tracings can now be done using computer software rather than being drawn by hand. Other radiographs used for diagnosis and treatment in orthodontics include:

- upper occlusals (used if the OPT is not clear in the upper incisor region)
- upper lateral occlusals
- peri-apicals
- postero-anterior (PA) skull.

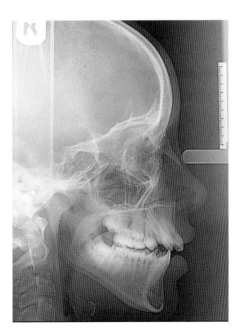

Figure 2.7 Example of cephalometric radiograph.
Source: Reproduced by kind permission of Jonathan Sandler.

The use of cone beam computed tomography, more routinely called cone beam CT, is becoming more widespread for orthodontic use (see Chapter 16 for examples). There is also the opportunity to take three-dimensional radiographs known as computed axial tomography scans, which can assist in producing computer-aided design/computer-aided manufacturing (CAD/CAM) models of the skull, maxilla and mandible, and three-dimensional facial soft tissue scans. These are often taken in conjunction with planning for orthognathic surgery and records.

Following clinical assessment and using the OPT and lateral skull radiograph, if required, the orthodontist can then formulate the treatment plan.

It is important to establish why the patient is seeking treatment as this will influence their keenness and compliance.

• are they themselves motivated (they want it for themselves)?
• are they being told they need it (they are trying to please someone else)?

With the X-ray films in hand, the orthodontist can then ask the patient and parent if they have any questions. These may include:

• the aim of orthodontic treatment
• how it is to be achieved
• what the treatment involves
• the best time for treatment to be done
• whether it is better to do the treatment in stages
• duration of treatment once started
• how many weeks between the appointments
• need for extractions as part of the treatment
• which appliance or sequence of appliances will be needed
• whether treatment will be painful or uncomfortable
• what type of retention will be needed and for how long it will need to be worn
• whether it will be possible to play sport (e.g. whether a mouthguard can be worn with a brace)
• whether it is possible to continue to play musical instruments by mouth (e.g. flute).

PHOTOGRAPHS

Photographs must only be taken with prior written consent from the patient or their parent/guardian. Patients can change their minds and remove consent at any time and they can also ask for a copy of the photographs taken.

The photographs can be taken in two ways:

• using a clinical camera with ring flash with details recorded in the patient's records and a photographic log book
• using a clinical camera with ring flash, with details recorded in the patient's records and the images stored and accessed on the computer.

Photographs must **never** be taken using a mobile phone or similar device.

If photographs are stored as a hard copy, they must be filed in either the patient's notes or hanging photo files. Photographs, like radiographs, are part of the patient's records. In either hard copy or digital format, these must be of good quality as they form part of the written clinical record. Clinical governance and good practice require that they must be stored securely to comply with current legislation concerning data protection. Everyone must comply with the current legislation concerning data protection regardless of where you work. Should guidance be needed, practices come under the Information Commissioners Office while hospital trusts will have their own data protection officers. There are strict protocols in place for the safe storage of images. A digital image can be enhanced when displayed on the computer screen but the original image must always be retained. Please see Chapter 23 for further information on encryption, etc.

The taking of photographs usually follows an established procedure that involves:

- a set position of each view required both intra- and extra-orally
- the number of photographs taken
- the same camera and background
- the same angles.

This ensures standardisation of all images taken.

Photographs should include extra-oral views, including facial views and profiles, and intra-oral views, using lip retractors. If there are any unusual areas of specific interest (e.g. traumatic bite), these must also be taken using photographic mouth mirrors.

Photographs are subsequently taken at the end of each stage of treatment, for example after rapid maxillary expansion and functional appliance therapy and then at the end of treatment. If the patient is undergoing orthognathic surgery, then more photographs are needed to record clinical changes and progress.

Some clinicians have access to a photographer, some take them themselves but the majority of orthodontic nurses are excellent photographers.

RISKS OF ORTHODONTIC TREATMENT

When assessing treatment options and the benefits that treatment will bring, the orthodontist will also advise the patient and parent/guardian of any possible risks that might occur. These risk factors are present in a minority of cases and some can easily be avoided (Figures 2.8 and 2.9).

Decalcification

Patients with poor oral hygiene can develop inflamed and unhealthy gums and may not be accepted for treatment. Patients who do not comply with oral hygiene instructions may experience decalcification/caries as a result of poor brushing, eating sweets and drinking fizzy drinks. The end result may be damaged teeth. In these cases the use of fluoride toothpastes and mouthwashes and mousse must be encouraged.

Failure to comply with oral hygiene may result in the early termination of treatment.

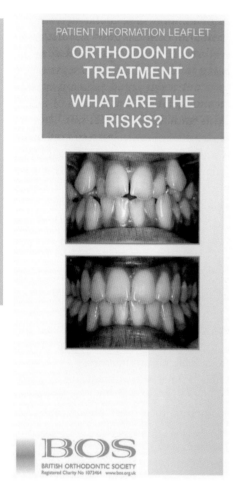

Figure 2.8 Leaflet on risks of orthodontic treatment. Source: Reproduced by kind permission of British Orthodontic Society.

Resorption

Sometimes, end-of-treatment radiographs show that there has been slight shortening of the roots on some teeth. This resorption happens during tooth movement. It is monitored and is rarely of significance but both patient and dentist need to be aware if it is significant for future dental reference. Teeth which have been previously damaged and teeth with thin roots are more prone to severe root resorption (Figure 2.10).

Relapse

This is the name given to tooth movement after completion of orthodontic treatment. Relapse can be caused by adverse growth or failure to comply with retainer wear.

Patient dissatisfaction

The patient feels that the aims and objectives set out during discussion of treatment were, in their opinion, not met.

(a)

(b)

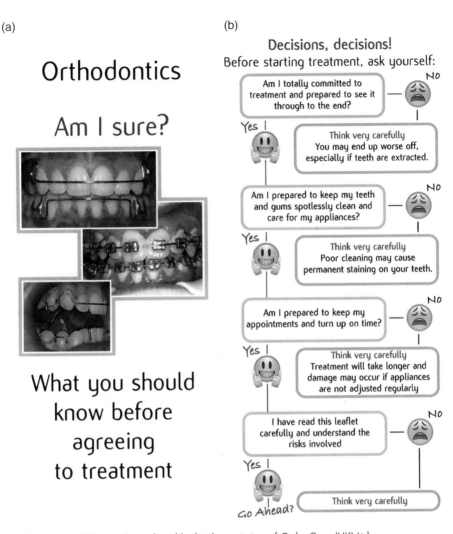

Figure 2.9 Am I sure? Source: Reproduced by kind permission of Ortho-Care (UK) Ltd.

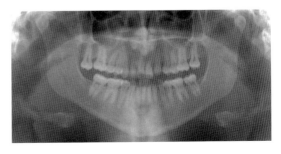

Figure 2.10 Radiograph showing resorption. Source: Reproduced by kind permission of Jonathan Sandler.

DISCUSSION AND CONSENT

Patients often have lots of questions and the orthodontic nurse is frequently the person they ask. It is at this time that the relationship starts to build between them. The nurse will get to know the patient over the course of the many visits and various procedures, and a friendly relaxed relationship will help to encourage their motivation and compliance. It is important that, as much as possible, the patient enjoys contributing and feeling part of their orthodontic journey.

It is important to remember that any baseline records taken:

- are legal documents
- help in diagnosis and treatment planning
- are needed for monitoring and scoring occlusal indices
- are needed for case presentations.

At a subsequent appointment the orthodontist, having looked at the models and radiographs, will formulate a treatment plan and then discuss this with the patient and their parent/or guardian and obtain informed consent.

If the patient is under the legal age of consent, then their parent or guardian usually gives informed consent. However, if the patient has full understanding of the proposed procedures, then they can consent themselves even if they are under 16 years of age (Figures 2.11 and 2.12).

Information leaflets may be given at this stage to be taken home and read.

TAKING BASELINE RECORDS

On the first appointment for treatment, the nurse needs to prepare:

- *the patient's clinical notes*
- *mouth mirror*
- *probe*
- *orthodontic ruler* (Figure 2.13)
- *hand mirror*
- *alginate, bowls and a spatula (vinyl polysiloxane can be used, but less likely when taking study models)*
- *impression trays*
- *wax (and bite registration recorder if used)*
- *wax knife*
- *method of softening wax (e.g. flame, blowtorch, hot water)*
- *glass of mouthwash and tissues*
- *laboratory sheet with instructions for technician*
- *solution to disinfect impressions*
- *camera (ring flash and digital)*
- *lip retractors* (Figure 2.14)
- *photographic mouth mirrors* (Figure 2.15), *if to be used*

Unit No: ....

NHS No: ....

Name: ....

CONSENT FOR AN INDIVIDUAL COURSE OF ORTHODONTIC TREATMENT

Treatment plan:

Benefits of treatment:

Risks of treatment (please see overleaf for more details):

☐ Permanent marks on teeth if not kept clean during treatment

☐ Shortening of the roots of teeth-occasionally this may be severe leading to tooth mobility or loss

☐ Discomfort

☐ Accidental swallowing of parts of brace requiring medical intervention

☐ Damage to nerve supply/ blood supply to individual teeth requiring root canal treatment

☐ Tooth movement after treatment if retainers not worn as advised

☐ Gum recession

☐ Other risks: ....
....
....

Patients should continue to see their family dentist for routine dental care during their orthodontic treatment

Information leaflets about orthodontic treatment have been provided as listed overleaf

Patient (or parent/ legal gardian)   **Clinician**

Signed ....   Signed ....

Print ....   Print ....

Date ....   Date ....

☐ Copy given to patient/ parent of legal guardian

Figure 2.11 Consent forms giving consent to orthodontic treatment. Source: Reproduced by kind permission of Jo Clark.

Information leaflets given:

☐ Keeping teeth and gums healthy (British Orthodontic Society)

☐ Fixed appliances (British Orthodontic Society)

☐ Removable appliances (British Orthodontic Society)

☐ Risks of treatment (British Orthodontic Society)

☐ Retainers (British Orthodontic Society)

☐ Functional appliances (British Orthodontic Society)

☐ Impacted canines (British Orthodontic Society)

☐ Brace-friendly food and drink (British Orthodontic Society)

☐ Interproximal reduction (British Orthodontic Society)

☐ Care of fixed appliances (Tepe)

☐ Other ....

Further information

Toothbrushing
It is essential that the teeth are kept clean and that the gums stay healthy during treatment. If toothbrushing is not kept up to standard during treatment, especially during fixed brace (train track) treatment, teeth can be permanently damaged leaving white or brown marks and possibly cavities where the brace has been. If toothbrushing is not kept up to standard during treatment then your orthodontist may advice that the brace should be removed before the teeth have been completely straightened.

Risks
1. Teeth can be damaged if toothbrushing is not up to standard (as above). A letter will be sent to you detailing how to keep your teeth and gums healthy after fixed braces are fitted
2. Discomfort: braces can be uncomfortable and your orthodontist will advice you about how to manage this eg. with painkillers and eating soft foods
3. Shortening of the teeth roots: The roots of the teeth will shorten as they are moved during treatment. This usually does not give problems but in a small percentage of patients it may be more severe and can lead to tooth mobility and loss. This cannot always be predicted but some people may be more susceptible and your orthodontist will discuss this you if they think you may be at increased risk.
4. Relapse: teeth will tend to move after treatment if retainers aren't worn as advised

Length of treatment
Your orthodontist will advice you about the likely length of treatment. Your treatment time will extend if your brace is broken frequently or if you miss your booked appoitments

Frequency of appointments
The teeth and braces need to be checked/ adjusted regularly (usually every 4-8 weeks). We cannot always guarantee appointments after school.

Failed and cancelled appointments
Poor or irregular attendance may lengthen the treatment and lead to a poorer result. If you need to change or cancel an appointment, please telephone xxxxxxxx

Stability of the treatment result
Most patients will be required to wear removable retainers part-time on a lifelong basis. Without retainers, teeth will tend to move. We will monitor your retainers for the first year after braces are removed. After this, we will write to your dentist to ask them to monitor your retainers. Your dentist will charge for new retainers when your retainers need replacement.

Figure 2.11 (*Continued*)

Unit No:	**Orthodontic Department**
NHS No:	**Clinical**
Surname:	**Photography/dental models**
Forenames:	**Consent Form**

This form is to be used to gain consent for taking pictures or making models of your teeth to enable clinical staff to assess your teeth and bite, monitor treatment progression and assess the outcome of your orthodontic treatment. These images/ dental models may be used for teaching purposes with your consent.

PATIENT SECTION

To comply with the Data Protection Act 2018, we need your permission before we take any photographs of you. Your health professional will have explained why they need to do this to best meet your health needs. If you have any further questions, please ask your health professional.

You have the right to change your mind at any time, including after you have signed this form.

PATIENT AGREEMENT

I understand the benefits and risks as described to me by my health professional.

I understand the recorded information will be used to support my (my child's)' treatment and I consent to the images/recordings being taken and stored safety with (my child's) health records.

I do/do not* give consent for these images (photos)/ dental models to be used for teaching purposes.

* delete as relevant

Name ....

Signature ....

Date ....

Full name of legal guardian if a child ....

Version 15.9.2018

Figure 2.12 Consent form giving consent to having dental photography. Source: Reproduced by kind permission of Jo Clark.

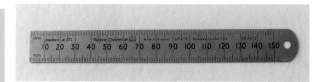

Figure 2.13 Orthodontic ruler. Source: Reproduced by kind permission of Ortho-Care (UK) Ltd.

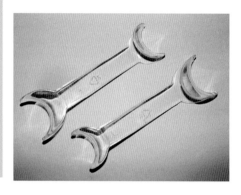

Figure 2.14 Lip retractors. Source: Reproduced by kind permission of TOC.

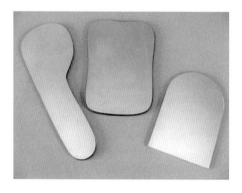

Figure 2.15 Photographic mouth mirrors. Source: Reproduced by kind permission of Ortho-Care (UK) Ltd.

- *information leaflets for the patient*
- *oral hygiene instruction leaflet for the patient.*

For the chairside procedure, the nurse ensures that:

- *the patient and staff wear personal protection*
- *the patient is seated comfortably*
- *a wax squash bite is taken to record the occlusion*
- *upper and lower alginate impressions are taken*
- *after disinfection, both impressions and bite are taken to the technician with instructions*
- *patient photographs are taken using lip and cheek retractors and photographic mirrors where appropriate.*

These photographic views should include:

- intra-oral:
  - left lateral
  - centric
  - right lateral
  - profile or lateral incisor view
- extra-oral:
  - full face (smiling)
  - full face (not smiling)
  - three-quarter view
  - profile (not smiling).

The nurse then:

- *gives the patient a leaflet on proposed treatment*
- *answers any further questions*
- *ensures that the patient has the correct series of appointments booked.*

Patients benefit from being given leaflets on their proposed treatment and on oral hygiene at this appointment because it gives them an opportunity to spend some time reading them before their next 'fitting' appointment. They can then get an idea of what will be happening when they come to start treatment.

ORTHODONTIC MODELS

Orthodontic study models can be obtained by taking either:

- alginate impressions, or
- a digital recording.

If the former, the study models must be boxed and a record made of the identification number and the patient's name. If the latter, then the scan must be securely stored on a computer system (Chapter 23 covers the storage of records in detail).

NB Orthodontic study models are reproductions of the dental arches and how they occlude together as they were on the day they were taken, and must always be marked with the patient's name and date when taken.

They are trimmed in a specific way, known as Angle's trimming. The upper model base does not have a rounded front, but is 'pointed' and angled. The lower model does have a rounded front (Figure 2.16).

Also, when the upper and lower models are trimmed together with the wax bite between them, it should be possible to:

- lay them on their backs or 'heels' (i.e. with the front teeth facing you) on a flat surface
- pick them up in the same position that you put them down
- make them stand without rocking and the teeth should stay together in the correct occlusion.

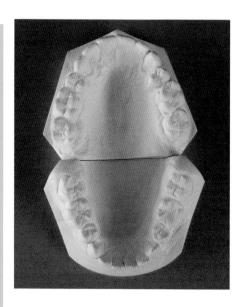

Figure 2.16 Example of trimmed orthodontic models.
Source: Reproduced by kind permission of Alan Hall.

Where records are taken digitally, please refer to Chapter 23.

Depending on the treatment plan, the patient is now ready:

- for the active treatment to begin and for an appliance to be fitted, *or*
- to undergo a period of watchful waiting, usually when there is a need to monitor adverse growth.

Chapter 3

Occlusal indices

Over the years the demand for orthodontic treatment has grown steadily. The public awareness of the condition and appearance of their teeth has driven the desire for 'straight teeth' and a confident smile. As a result of this, more and more patients are asking to be referred, or referring themselves, for orthodontic treatment.

The Index of Orthodontic Treatment Need (IOTN), devised by Dr Stephen Richmond, Dr Kevin O'Brien, Mr Iain Buchanan and Mr Donald Burden, incorporates an aesthetic and dental health component as a scale for standardising measurement by including:

- degree of severity of the malocclusion
- aesthetics.

The increasing demand for treatment may mean that not all patients who would like treatment are eligible to receive it under a third party-funded system such as the National Health Service (NHS).

Where there are finite resources, there has to be a balance between what is desired and what is needed. This means prioritising treatment and takes into account:

- the entry levels for treatment
- availability of funds and operators
- the hierarchy of treatment providers.

To assess the needs of a patient using a standard set of criteria means that each orthodontic assessment arrives at a similar conclusion. As such, it needs to have several functions, which involve:

- an assessment that uses a series of benchmark criteria
- measurement of the severity of the presenting conditions
- assessment of whether by treating their orthodontic problem the patient would have significant benefits.

IOTN has several components.

Basic Guide to Orthodontic Dental Nursing, Second Edition. Fiona Grist.
© 2020 John Wiley & Sons Ltd. Published 2020 by John Wiley & Sons Ltd.

DENTAL HEALTH COMPONENT

This measures and quantifies the severity of the malocclusion in categories that range from IOTN 5, the most severe, to IOTN 1, where there is no significant deviation from normal (Figure 3.1).

In any malocclusion, the worst deviations from the norm are measured. These may include:

- supernumerary teeth
- impacted teeth
- a reverse overjet
- displacement of teeth
- severe rotations
- crossbites
- hypodontia (missing teeth)
- an increased overjet.

The dental health ruler (Figure 3.2) is helpful for maintaining a consistent method of taking measurements. It prioritises, in descending order:

- M – missing teeth
- O – overjet
- C – crossbite
- D – displaced contact points
- O – open/overbite.

Many clinicians also use these findings for audit purposes.

The dental health ruler is a small clear scale for measuring the occlusal features on study models. The scores documented on pre- and post-treatment models gauge the level of effectiveness, which is recorded as:

- greatly improved
- moderately improved
- little or no improvement.

AESTHETIC COMPONENT

This shows the appearance of the teeth – what the patient looks like. It comprises a sheet of 10 photographs showing increasing severity of malocclusion (Figure 3.3). These photos are all the same size, are produced in colour and are anterior views of the teeth in occlusion. They range from 1 (no irregularities, an acceptable occlusion) to 10 (severe irregularities where the malocclusion is in greater need of treatment).

The 10-point rating scale was first published in 1987 by Ruth Evans and William Shaw.

TABLE 1   THE DENTAL HEALTH COMPONENT
           OF THE INDEX OF ORTHODONTIC TREATMENT NEED (IOTN)

GRADE 5 (Need treatment)

5.i   Impeded eruption of teeth (except for third molars) due to crowding, displacement, the presence of supernumerary teeth, retained deciduous teeth and any pathological cause.

5.h   Extensive hypodontia with restorative implications (more than 1 tooth missing in any quadrant) requiring pre-restorative orthodontics.

5.a   Increased overjet greater than 9mm.

5.m   Reverse overjet greater than 3.5min with reported masticatory and speech difficulties.

5.p   Defects of cleft lip and palate and other craniofacial anomalies.

5.s   Submerged deciduous teeth.

GRADE 4 (Need treatment)

4.h   Less extensive hypodontia requiring prerestorative orthodontics or orthodontic space closure to obviate the need for a prosthesis.

4.a   Increased overjet greater than 6mm but less than or equal to 9mm.

4.b   Reverse overjet greater than 3.5mm with no masticatory or speech difficulties.

4.m   Reverse overjet greater than 1mm but less than 3.5mm with recorded masticatory and speech difficulties.

4.c   Anterior or posterior crossbites with greater than 2mm discrepancy between retruded contact position and intercuspal position.

4.1   Posterior lingual crossbite with no functional occlusal contact in one or both buccal segments.

4.d   Severe contact point displacements greater than 4mm.

4.e   Extreme lateral or anterior open bites greater than 4mm.

4.f   Increased and complete overbite with gingival or palatal trauma.

4.t   Partially erupted teeth, tipped and impacted against adjacent teeth.

4.x   Presence of supernumery teeth.

GRADE 3 (Borderline need)

3.a   Increased overjet greater than 3.5mm but less than or equal to 6mm. with incompetent lips.

3.b   Reverse overjet greater than 1mm but less than or equal to 3.5mm.

3.c   Anterior or posterior crossbites with greater than 1mm but less than or equal to 2mm discrepancy between retruded contact position and intercuspal position.

3.d   Contact point displacements greater than 2mm but less than or equal to 4mm.

3.e   Lateral or anterior open bite greater than 2mm but less than or equal to 4mm.

3.f   Deep overbite complete on gingival or palatal tissues but no trauma.

GRADE 2 (Little)

2.a   Increased overjet greater than 3.5mm but less than or equal to 6mm with competent lips.

2.b   Reverse overjet greater than 0mm but less than or equal to 1mm.

2.c   Anterior or posterior crossbite with less than or equal to 1mm discrepancy between retruded contact position and intercuspal position.

2.d   Contact point dispalcements greater than 1mm but less than or equal to 2mm.

2.e   Anterior or posterior openbite greater than 1mm but less than or equal to 2mm

2.f   Increased overbite greater than or equal 3.5mm without gingival contact.

2.g   Pre-normal or post-normal occlusions with no other anomalies (includes up to half a unit discrepancy).

GRADE 1 (None)

1.   Extremely minor malocussions including contact point displacements less than 1mm.

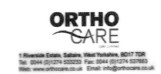

1 Riverside Estate, Saltaire, West Yorkshire, BD17 7DR
Tel: 0044 (0)1274 533233 Fax: 0044 (0)1274 537663
Web: www.orthocare.co.uk Email: info@orthocare.co.uk

Figure 3.1 Dental health component. Source: Reproduced by kind permission of Ortho-Care (UK) Ltd. © University of Manchester.

OCCLUSAL INDICES

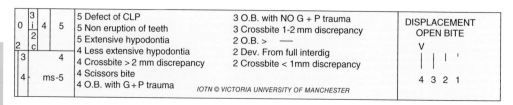

3				5 Defect of CLP	3 O.B. with NO G + P trauma	DISPLACEMENT
0	i	4	5	5 Non eruption of teeth	3 Crossbite 1-2 mm discrepancy	OPEN BITE
2	2			5 Extensive hypodontia	2 O.B. > —	
	c			4 Less extensive hypodontia	2 Dev. From full interdig	V
3			4	4 Crossbite > 2 mm discrepancy	2 Crossbite < 1mm discrepancy	
4		ms-5		4 Scissors bite		4 3 2 1
				4 O.B. with G + P trauma *IOTN © VICTORIA UNIVERSITY OF MANCHESTER*		

Figure 3.2 IOTN dental health component ruler (disposable). Source: Reproduced by kind permission of Ortho-Care (UK) Ltd. © University of Manchester.

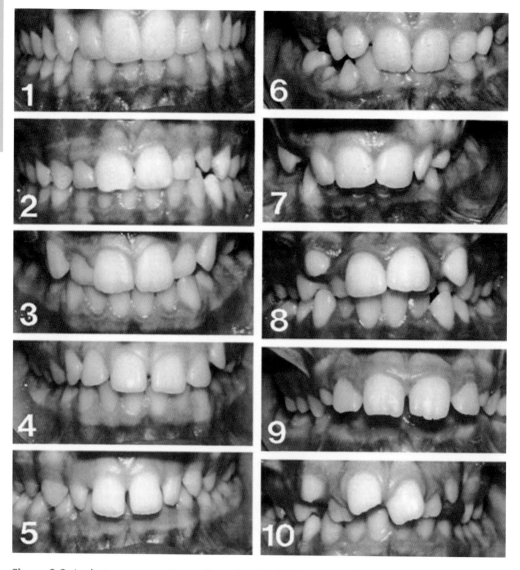

Figure 3.3 Aesthetic component. Source: Reproduced by kind permission of Professor Steven Richmond and Ortho-Care (UK) Ltd. © University of Manchester.

THE PAR INDEX

The Peer Assessment Rating (PAR) index was formulated by a group of specialist orthodontists to record the dental malocclusion at any developmental stage. It uses precise criteria to provide a quantitative objective method for measuring malocclusion and the efficacy of treatment using pre- and post-treatment study models. This is becoming a much more widespread practice as it is often required as part of contract monitoring in primary care. While some clinicians use independent laboratories to score their cases, many more are doing it in-house by members of their dental team.

Scores are applied to several different occlusal traits that make up the malocclusion. The individual scores are summed to obtain a total that represents the degree that the case deviates from normal occlusion and alignment. The score of zero indicates good alignment and higher scores (rarely over 50) indicate increased levels of irregularity. The difference between the pre- and post-treatment PAR scores indicates the degree of improvement as a result of orthodontic intervention.

The PAR ruler has been designed to make all measurements easier. The information on the ruler summarises the index and allows quick assessments. The top three sections (Figure 3.4) provide a short-hand summary of buccal occlusion. Antero-posterior, transverse and vertical scores are summed for each buccal segment. The next section summarises centreline rating, which is recorded in relation to lower incisor width. The overbite section allows recording of overlap in relation to coverage of the lower incisors. Open bite is recorded with reference to the length of the lines to the right. In the contact point displacement section, the length of the line is matched to the contact point displacements. If the distance between the contact points is greater than the line, the higher rating applies. Contact point displacements are summed for each anterior segment. The final section summarises overjet and anterior crossbite ratings. These ratings are summed if both are present.

There are five components of the PAR index (Table 3.1) and each is discussed in the following sections.

Anterior segments

Scores are recorded for both upper and lower anterior segment alignment. The recording zone is from the mesial contact of the canine on one side to the mesial contact point of the canine on the opposite side. The features recorded are crowding and impacted teeth (Table 3.2). Contact point displacement is recorded as the shortest distance between the contact points of adjacent teeth parallel to the occlusal plane. The greater the contact point displacement, the greater the score.

Impactions of incisors and canines are recorded. A tooth is regarded as impacted if the space between the two adjacent teeth is less than or equal to 4 mm. Both ectopic incisors and canines are recorded in the anterior segment. Scores for the contact point placements and impacted/ectopic teeth are summed to give an overall score for each anterior segment.

If there is potential crowding in the mixed dentition, average mesio-distal widths are used to calculate the space deficiency (Table 3.3). If the space remaining for an unerupted tooth is 4 mm or less, then an impaction is recorded in the anterior segment.

OCCLUSAL INDICES

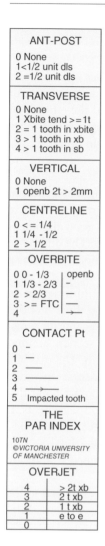

ANT-POST

0 None
1 <1/2 unit dls
2 =1/2 unit dls

TRANSVERSE

0 None
1 Xbite tend >= 1t
2 = 1 tooth in xbite
3 > 1 tooth in xb
4 > 1 tooth in sb

VERTICAL

0 None
1 openb 2t > 2mm

CENTRELINE

0 < = 1/4
1 1/4 - 1/2
2 > 1/2

OVERBITE

0 0 - 1/3	openb
1 1/3 - 2/3	–
2 > 2/3	—
3 >= FTC	—
4	→—

CONTACT Pt

0 –
1 —
2 —
3 ——
4 →—
5 Impacted tooth

THE PAR INDEX

10TN
©VICTORIA UNIVERSITY
OF MANCHESTER

OVERJET

4	> 2t xb
3	2 t xb
2	1 t xb
1	e to e
0	

Figure 3.4 PAR index ruler (disposable). Abbreviations: xbite, xb, crossbite; sb, scissor bite; open b, open bite; FTC, full tooth coverage; t, tooth/teeth; e to e, edge to edge; tend, tendency; 1/2 unit dis, half unit discrepancy (cusp to cusp). Source: Reproduced by kind permission of Ortho-Care (UK) Ltd. © University of Manchester.

Table 3.1 Components of the PAR index.

Upper and lower anterior segments
Left and right buccal occlusion
Overjet
Overbite
Centreline

Buccal occlusion

The buccal occlusion is recorded for both left and right sides. The fit of the teeth is recorded in all three planes. The recording zone is from the canine to the last molar, either first, second or third. All features are recorded when the teeth are in occlusion. The antero-posterior, vertical and transverse scores are summed for each buccal segment (Table 3.4).

Table 3.2 Contact point displacement scores.

Score	Displacement
1	0–1 mm
2	1.1–2 mm
3	4.1–8 mm
4	> 8 mm
5	Impacted teeth

Table 3.3 Mixed dentition crowding assessment using average mesio-distal widths.

Upper		
Canine	8 mm	Total = 22 mm (impaction ≤ 18 mm)
First premolar	7 mm	
Second premolar	7 mm	
Lower		
Canine	7 mm	Total = 21 mm (impaction ≤ 17 mm)
First premolar	7 mm	
Second premolar	7 mm	

Table 3.4 Buccal occlusion scores.

Antero-posterior
0   Good interdigitation
Class I, II or III
1   Less than ½ unit from full interdigitation
2   ½ unit (cusp to cusp)

Vertical
0   No open bite
1   Lateral open bite on at least two teeth > 2 mm

Transverse
0   No crossbite
1   Crossbite tendency
2   Single tooth in crossbite
3   More than one tooth in crossbite
4   More than one tooth in scissor bite

Temporary developmental stages and submerging deciduous teeth are excluded.

Overjet

Positive overjet as well as anterior teeth in crossbite are recorded (Table 3.5). The recording zone includes all incisor teeth. The most prominent incisor overjet is identified and the overjet is recorded to the labial aspect of the incisal edge. When recording the overjet, the ruler is held parallel to the occlusal plane and radial to the line of the arch. It is not uncommon to see two upper laterals in crossbite as well as an increased overjet on the central incisors. In this situation, if the overjet was 4 mm, the score would be 3 for the crossbite and 1 for the positive overjet (= 4 in total).

Table 3.5 Overjet assessment.

Overjet
0   0–3 mm
1   3.1–5 mm
2   5.1–7 mm
3   7.1–9 mm
4   >9 mm

Anterior crossbites
0   No crossbite
1   One or more teeth edge to edge
2   One single tooth in crossbite
3   Two teeth in crossbite
4   More than two teeth in crossbite

Canine crossbites are recorded in the overjet assessment.

Table 3.6 Overbite assessment.

Open bite
0   No open bite
1   Open bite ≤ 1 mm
2   Open bite 1.1–2 mm
3   Open bite 2.1–3 mm
4   Open bite ≥ 4 mm

Overbite
0   Less than or equal to one-third coverage of the lower incisor
1   Greater than one-third but less than two-thirds coverage of the lower incisor
2   Greater than two-thirds coverage of the lower incisor
3   Greater than or equal to full tooth coverage

Table 3.7 Centreline assessment.

0   Coincident and up to one-quarter lower incisor width
1   One-quarter to one-half lower incisor width
2   Greater than one-half lower incisor width

Overbite

Records the worst vertical overlap or open bite of any of the four incisors. Open bite is recorded in relation to the coverage of the lower incisors or the degree of open bite (Table 3.6).

Centreline assessment

The difference between the upper and lower dental midlines is recorded in relation to the lower dental midline (Table 3.7).

ICON

The Index of Complexity, Outcome and Need (ICON) is a development from IOTN and also includes the complexity of treatment.

MANAGEMENT

Under the NHS, referrals may go through a referral management service and are allocated the orthodontic operators by commissioners. These are sent to either:

- primary care, i.e. specialist orthodontic practices, or
- secondary care, i.e. hospital services.

In order to qualify for funding:

- in primary care, the patient needs to have an IOTN rating of 3.6 or above
- in secondary care, the patient's score must be 4 or 5.

NHS commissioners may have an appeals procedure for dealing with patients whose score puts them in the low-priority category but who are still considered in need of orthodontic treatment by their dentist or orthodontist.

The IOTN ensures that the same criteria are universally used.

Note: All products relating to the occlusal indices standards are the copyright of the University of Manchester. Ortho-Care (UK) Ltd. acts as the sole distributor for the products and pays a royalty to the university for the privilege. They are reproduced here by their kind permission.

OCCLUSAL INDICES

Chapter 4
Motivation

In general, patients who are undergoing orthodontic treatment are quite enthusiastic about their treatment. Maintaining this enthusiasm can be difficult, but it truly is the secret of success.

Orthodontic treatment involving fixed appliance therapy takes:

- on average 18–24 months
- regular visits.

The optimum time to do this is in the early second dentition.

For a young patient, perception of time is quite unlike that of their orthodontist or parents/guardians. They live in a world of no waiting, touch-of-a-button, on demand, instant results. Most young patients see a school term as ages and the time between one birthday and the next is off the scale. So, the start of treatment is probably the keenest they are going to be.

Orthodontic treatment is like preparing a garden: you plant and wait patiently until the flowers appear but sometimes have a long period before you can see any signs of progress. Sometimes, in the early stages, when the hoped-for 'instant fix' is just not happening, the patient becomes despondent when no visible change is seen.

When this stage is reached, there are often tell-tale signs:

- oral hygiene starts to deteriorate
- there are breakages
- there are occasional missed appointments
- the patient can become uncommunicative, even sullen.

This is where motivation has to be rekindled.

Unlike patients in general practice, orthodontic patients:

- are referred in from their regular dentist
- are seen for a course of treatment and retention
- not routinely seen again.

During orthodontic treatment, patients are seen on average every 4–6 weeks. During that time you get to know them and their parents quite well. Sometimes they may have had a

Basic Guide to Orthodontic Dental Nursing, Second Edition. Fiona Grist.
© 2020 John Wiley & Sons Ltd. Published 2020 by John Wiley & Sons Ltd.

brother or sister in treatment before them so that both the parents and new patient will be familiar with the surgery and the routine of appliance adjustment appointments.

Many have friends at school who are undergoing the same treatment and may be coping with similar experiences. This can be helpful if it is constructive, and not being the only one with a brace helps. There is often discussion of treatments between patients, especially at school. Like all chatter:

- there are those who tell tales of doom and gloom
- others who tease
- but on rare occasions, banter may become bullying.

If this happens, parents and schools must get involved. It must be stopped.

When orthodontic patients are assessed, the amount of support they will receive is important. The best-case scenario is a keen patient with a keen parent. The worst-case scenario is a patient who has no concerns but has been encouraged to have treatment. These reluctant patients look you right in the eye with a stare that says:

- 'just you see who is the boss'
- 'I will have the last word'.

It is the beginning of an uphill struggle, often littered with breakages and lost appliances along the way!

When the nurse builds rapport with a patient, it is easier to know what motivates them. As the treatment progresses the patient experiences a mixture of:

- seeing the benefits appearing
- wanting the braces removed as soon as possible.

There needs to be a steady stream of encouragement at this stage.

Often for the younger patient, visual encouragement in the form of a sticker helps. It is surprising what the motivational power of a sticker can achieve.

Keep reinforcing and encouraging the positives, such as:

- *how good the teeth are looking already*
- *show them the start models ('Look how far we have come!!')*
- *remind them what they looked like before treatment*
- *emphasise how much of the hard work is already done*
- *try to have a provisional deband date to aim for, e. g. off before the school prom or they go on holiday*
- *keep praising the positive and cajole on all the negative areas.*

The best motivation comes from the patient themselves, but when they hear you say **'You are doing SO well, what a star'**, *the smile you get tells you that together you will get there.*

If the oral hygiene is in the doldrums:

- *show photos of results that poor cleaning might bring*
- *give them a new type of interspace brush*
- *give them a couple of tubes of different toothpaste*
- *try getting them to use disclosing tablets.*

MOTIVATION

If they are wearing elastomerics (O-rings), encourage them to make their own choice of colours. This can give them back ownership of the appliance, pride in their efforts and achievement in undergoing the therapy.

Sometimes, empowering patients gets good results, for example if they need to keep a diary or log of their participation in treatment. You are, in effect, asking them to provide information about themselves. You are not reinforcing what they need to do; they are affirming that they know what to do.

Asking them to keep a 'food diary', use a sticker or emoji progress chart, or 'trial' which type of interspace brush or toothpaste they find most effective can make them proactive. For some patients this focuses them and they take ownership of the actions. For younger patients, never underestimate the motivating power of a sticker or emoji, because this is a 'travelling leaflet', a written endorsement of how well you think they are doing.

At the deband appointment, admire, admire and admire again!

Nature helps us here, as most teenage patients present with:

- malaligned, often protruding teeth
- many problems associated with hormonal teenagers.

However, by the deband date there are huge improvements on all fronts and the 'ugly duckling' patient who began treatment has been transformed into a confident swan.

There is nothing to compare with the look of absolute delight when the sometimes awkward, rebellious, monosyllabic teenager of a couple of years ago looks in the mirror and sees the changes. You have come to know them, their highs and lows, what music they listen to, their sports, their clothes, what's going on in their lives, and sometimes their anxieties and concerns. It is quite amazing just how much you do get to know about them.

Their treatment is like a journey you have travelled together. As a nurse you have helped when their enthusiasm flagged, when the temptation to eat everything that is banned overtook them, so you are part of their success. A great result for them is a great result for you as well. For orthodontic nurses, this special relationship with the patient you know for such a relatively short time is one of the main differences between nursing in orthodontics and general practice.

However, it is not all over yet. With the malocclusion corrected and the teeth aligned, we are about to enter the retention phase.

RETENTION

The majority of patients wear their retainers as and when asked, and have no problems (Figure 4.1).

However, for a few patients the feeling is that:

- they have finished treatment
- their braces have been removed
- there are no more monthly appointments to keep.

With straight teeth, their mission is accomplished.

MOTIVATION

MOTIVATION

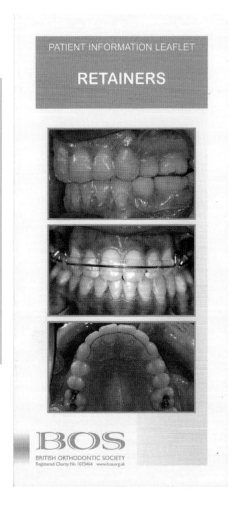

Figure 4.1 Retainers leaflet. Source: Reproduced by kind permission of British Orthodontic Society.

Patients are always told that teeth after debanding can (and will) move if the retainers are not worn. However, a few patients think that this is something that happens to other people. They decide when and how to wear their retainers, hoping that it will probably be enough to get them through.

Alas not.

It is not a matter of 'will the teeth move' but 'how far will they go' (Figure 4.2) Relapse is disappointing for everyone involved. Retention really is one of the hardest stages with which to get the patient to comply. They may have reacted well to 'compliance' whilst in active treatment because they were regularly encouraged and reminded.

Motivation is not the same. You can get a patient who is not self-motivated to comply – they just do what is asked of them. However, once you are out of sight and, for them, out of mind, it is then down to the individual to encourage themselves, to be self-motivating and regulate themselves. These patients often develop a very relaxed attitude to wearing their retainers.

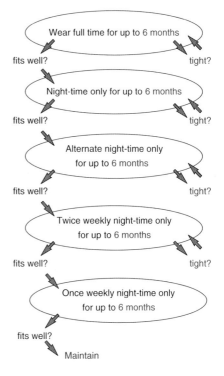

Figure 4.2 Inside a Retainer Leaflet. Source: Reproduced by kind permission of Ortho-Care (UK) Ltd.

For whatever reason some patients will return to the surgery many months (often years) after their braces were removed, with teeth a long way from where they were on the day they were debanded. Nine times out of ten, away from the regular visits to the surgery, the motivation to wear the retainers was no match for the 'I'll risk it, it will be OK' hopefuls. A few are lucky and get away with it; many more are not.

So, at the retainer fitting appointment:

- *tell your patients how great they look*
- *compare their teeth now with their initial models and photos*
- *warn them that Nature will fight back, given half a chance*
- *empower them to follow the regime for wearing their retainers*
- *tell them it is really important*
- *tell them not to risk undoing all the hard work they, and everyone else, put in and keep enjoying the great smile they have got now.*

PATIENTS WHO ARE MOTIVATED AND READILY COMPLY

The needs of adult patients who come for treatment may vary, from correcting mild over-crowding to completely rehabilitating that individual's occlusion. Whatever their malocclusion may be, it is a concern to them. For these patients especially, the improvement in their appearance, and often function, will boost their self-esteem.

Some patients have lived, and been unhappy, with their problem for a long time. This group of patients has a high level of compliance and a great deal of self-motivation. However, while patient motivation is vital, of equal importance is the motivation of the individual members of the orthodontic team.

The orthodontic team

Motivated staff perform well. They are:

* proactive
* happy in their work
* positive
* efficient.

In short, they are empowered.

Orthodontists have long acknowledged their nursing staff to be 'key' members of a highly specialised and productive team. Every individual in the team has a role to play and recognises how they rely on one another. Once established, trust within a team ensures valuable co-operation as well, and when the need arises, to solve problems and resolve issues.

Accepting and sharing responsibility is a strong motivator. When team members are empowered:

* it reflects in their work
* they become more productive
* they are excellent ambassadors for their practice/department/unit.

Motivation in the team setting can come from above, sideways and below.

Above
> From the clinicians who:

* involve and encourage their nurses to learn more
* delegate responsibilities
* develop their potential
* provide continuing professional development (CPD).

Sideways
> From colleagues:

* other nurses in the surgeries
* reception and clerical staff, managers
* technicians

- ones you meet at conferences or meetings
- people who get you interested in what new things they are doing
- networking.

Below

- nurses who have just started in your workplace and need training and encouragement
- nurses who are learning new techniques and need demonstrations to give them an extra skill
- nurses that you are mentoring and who need support.

If you are motivated yourself, you lead by example. When motivating their patients, orthodontic nurses and therapists are in a league of their own.

- motivation is enthusiasm
- empowerment fuels enthusiasm
- enthusiasm develops the individual.

MOTIVATION

Chapter 5
Leaflets

Leaflets are written communication – either advice or instruction – that are given to the patient.

Orthodontic treatment is complex and patients need to play their part in looking after and adjusting their appliances where necessary.

For patients and their parent/guardian, an important part of being able to comply with what is being asked of them is to fully understand:

- exactly what it is they need to do
- why they are doing it
- what they are aiming to achieve.

In order to do that there must be good communication between the patient and the clinical dental staff.

Therefore, we need to create trust between the orthodontic team and the patient:

- to persuade and influence them to carry out the instructions
- impress on them their role in getting the best result at the end of treatment.

Leaflets given to patients should cover two areas.

- Information: what the treatment entails, what the patients can expect, etc.
- Instruction: their contribution to the treatment, what they need to do, etc.

There are many leaflets available and the orthodontic nurse needs to select the most appropriate for each situation. The most commonly used leaflets are the ones that you give to patients. This book provides examples of a variety of styles.

The British Orthodontic Society produces many excellent leaflets for patients as well as advice and clinical guidance for the orthodontic team (Figure 5.1). These include:

- advice on digit/dummy sucking
- orthodontic management of the medically compromised patient
- advice on the use of headgear and facebows
- use and storage of digital photographs
- orthodontic records (collection and management)
- advice on providing treatment for wind instrumentalists
- dental nurse competencies in orthodontic practice.

Basic Guide to Orthodontic Dental Nursing, Second Edition. Fiona Grist.
© 2020 John Wiley & Sons Ltd. Published 2020 by John Wiley & Sons Ltd.

These are a few of the many leaflets that cover a wide and diverse range of subjects. They are useful for the orthodontic nurse to read and to update on current best practice. By visiting http://www.bos-org.uk you can learn more about the subjects and titles available.

When verbal instructions are given to a patient it is often:

- at the end of a procedure which has been tiring for them
- when they may be anxious
- when they may feel stressed about how strange the appliance feels
- when they, and their parents, are glad that having the consultation/procedure is nearly over.

Sometimes neither the patient nor their accompanying adult is fully listening to what is being said, but are just listening for, and focused on, an aspect of concern to them, perhaps the word 'injection' or 'headgear'.

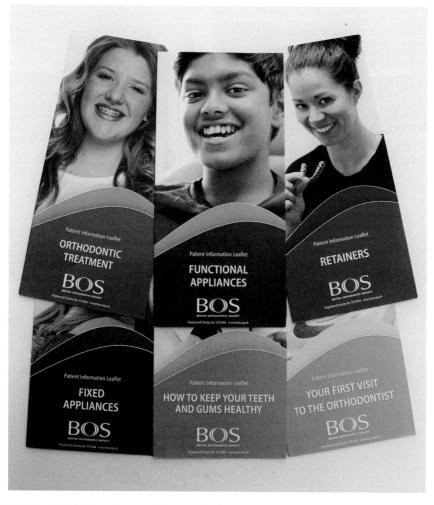

Figure 5.1 British Orthodontic Society information leaflets. Source: Reproduced by kind permission of the British Orthodontic Society.

When trying to get information across to patients it has been estimated that:

- only 7% of communication is verbal
- 38% is passed on by the speed and tone of voice
- the main part, a massive 55%, of the message is delivered visually.

What the patient sees, be it body language or eye contact, engages his or her attention. They will always remember how they felt when you spoke to them but not always what you said. Anxiety is a barrier to listening and understanding.

So, with this in mind, after the patient has been given advice and instructions verbally by the nurse, it is really beneficial that they are given a printed instruction leaflet as well. The patient takes this home and can go back to it when they are not under pressure and can understand the information more effectively. Given that the majority of patients are young, it is also better to repeat information that they may have forgotten rather than assume they know it, so ending up with a problem.

However, we are all different and choose what we read in a style that we like and which feels comfortable. This is a personal preference and is not a 'one size fits all', so several formats are available. They all carry the same message but while some may feature more cartoon-like drawings, others may be set out in a question and answer format. Others may consist of little individual bites of information, not part of a text. It doesn't matter what form the information takes, as long as it is read (Figure 5.2).

When a patient has the new patient consultation appointment sent to them, it is helpful to enclose the leaflet 'Your first visit to the orthodontist' (Figure 5.3). This leaflet outlines what is likely to happen and what will be discussed. For many patients the thought of this visit is quite worrying, and for some children who have not had any experience of dental treatment (e.g. fillings) they don't know what to expect. Their peers at school often take advantage of this anxiety, tell them gruesome stories and generally 'wind them up'. Often this can add to their stress. Some patients even worry that treatment will start straight away and their teeth could be taken out there and then! They can experience the same feelings that an adult has when going for an interview or taking their driving test.

One of the symptoms of this stress is not listening or rather just listening for certain words, such as 'pain', 'problems with speech', 'altered appearance' and worst of all 'extractions'. So if patients know what is likely to happen they may not be totally relaxed but the reassuring information in the leaflet goes a long way to helping them get a good night's sleep, and to be able to eat their breakfast before they arrive in the chair. This makes them more receptive to listening and understanding what is being said.

Leaflets are also given at the beginning of each phase of treatment, in order to:

- always reinforce the verbal messages
- tell the patient the aims of treatment
- explain how it will affect them
- indicate what type of braces they will need
- advise how to best cope with them
- provide guidance how to look after and clean them.

In addition, leaflets can have the names of the nurses they will meet when they have their first appointment and during any treatment. This can foster a more personal relationship rather than there being a lot of new faces in unfamiliar surroundings talking in a strange orthodontic language.

LEAFLETS

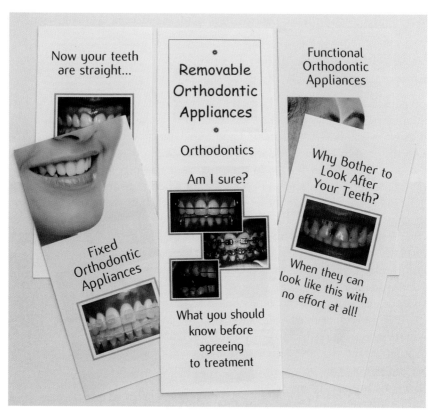

Figure 5.2 Ortho-Care information leaflet. Source: Reproduced by kind permission of Ortho-Care (UK) Ltd.

The leaflet also provides contact numbers. This encourages patients to feel that, should there be anything about which they are unsure, a quick phone call to the surgery for clarification will be better than worrying unnecessarily and giving the molehill a chance to become a mountain. If you ask patients at the end of treatment what it was that they found most scary when they came for their first appointment, the answers will often surprise you. The more problems you can eliminate, the easier it will be.

Given that patients find the prospect of orthodontic treatment daunting and can become stressed and anxious, explanation and empathy can help this. Most importantly, the nurse can often pass on to the orthodontist anything which is specially worrying a patient, acting as their mouthpiece, often broaching a subject or asking a question for them. In this way patients, or their parents/guardians, will feel able to mention concerns that they think are silly or minor, but which are causing genuine anxiety.

Good leaflets are in colour, with informative, easy to understand text and clear photographic images. If there is any apprehension concerning treatment, it is often helpful to give the patient the leaflet beforehand. In this way they can get used to the idea and 'get their head round it' so that it is not an unknown quantity. It is the patients with the unknown to deal with that their friends find so easy to make scared.

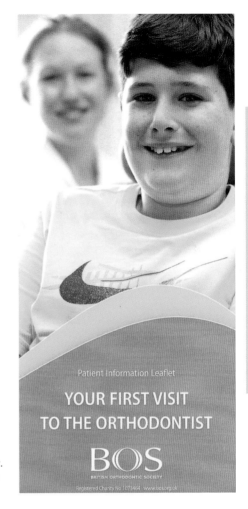

Figure 5.3 'Your first visit to the orthodontist' leaflet. Source: Reproduced by kind permission of the British Orthodontic Society.

There are very many styles and types of leaflets available. Clinical subjects covered include:

- fixed appliances
- removable appliances
- functional appliances
- extra-oral traction
- retainers
- mini screws
- oral hygiene.

While some are produced by professional bodies such as the British Orthodontic Society or by orthodontic supply companies (e.g. Ortho-Care), others are commercially produced to enhance or endorse a product. These are produced in a different style.

Many practices and individuals design and produce their own leaflets. These are often created in-house as a combined effort by all the staff of a practice or department. These in-house leaflets can be really helpful if they include extra information that covers emergency details, e. g. what patients need to do if they have a problem. This information includes hours when the surgeries are open, a 'who's who' of staff, details of whom to contact and the telephone number in an emergency. This can be reassuring for patients and leaflets containing such information are often stored at home in a safe place 'just in case'.

Chapter 6

Oral hygiene

The majority of patients wearing orthodontic appliances are teenagers and as a group they are always hungry and need regular intakes of food. They tend to snack between meals and very often after an appliance is fitted the wise words on the dietary sheet given to them in the surgery are forgotten or ignored when the tummy rumbles between meals or temptation, in the disguise of a hard, sticky or crunchy snack, is put in their path. Either way, the suggestions on the advice sheet fly from their thoughts as the food goes into their mouths.

The oral hygiene leaflet should be a way of helping patients to help themselves, to maximise all the effort they put in by doing the right things in the right order. If they do this, they minimise the danger of permanently damaging their teeth by decalcification, erosion and decay.

So, how effective is an oral hygiene leaflet and how do you as an orthodontic dental nurse get your patients to take the advice on board?

FOR REMOVABLE APPLIANCES

Removable braces have acrylic baseplates which can trap food between them and:

- the palate
- the lips
- the tongue.

Patients are advised after every meal (and snack!) to:

- remove the appliance and clean it under running water, using regular toothpaste
- do this over a sink full of water (should the appliance slip out of the patient's hand, it will not shatter on the basin)
- clean their teeth thoroughly
- clean their palate and gums, taking extra care around the gum margins
- once a week soak the appliance in a cleaner such as Retainer Brite, which is designed especially for the purpose (Figure 6.1).

Basic Guide to Orthodontic Dental Nursing, Second Edition. Fiona Grist.
© 2020 John Wiley & Sons Ltd. Published 2020 by John Wiley & Sons Ltd.

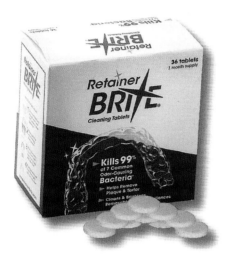

Figure 6.1 Retainer Brite for cleaning removable appliances. Source: Reproduced by kind permission of Ortho-Care (UK) Ltd.

Essix® retainers

This type of retainer should be rinsed under running water; if necessary a soft toothbrush can be used with liquid soap but never toothpaste. Toothpaste is abrasive and the retainer will become scratched, making it look dull and cloudy.

Aligners

Aligners must also be rinsed in cold water and cleaned with a soft brush and liquid soap if necessary; never use toothpaste. No appliance can be self-cleansing and trapped food debris can irritate the soft tissues of the mouth, which can become inflamed.

FOR FIXED APPLIANCES

Fixed appliances are not the easiest to keep clean, but the consequence of not doing so is teeth that are permanently marked or decayed. Straight but marked teeth is not a good look and certainly not one that patients want. Try to impress on patients that these are **their** teeth they are damaging. It is their responsibility!

Besides regular tooth brushing, and flossing (if possible), the orthodontic patient has to be extra careful with:

- hard, sticky or crunchy foods
- sweets or crisps between meals
- fizzy or cola drinks
- chewing gum
- fresh fruit juice (especially if drunk between meals).

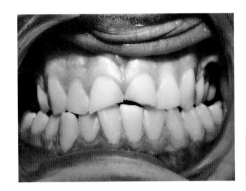

Figure 6.2 Incisal erosion due to fizzy drinks drunk from a can. Source: Reproduced by kind permission of Alan Hall.

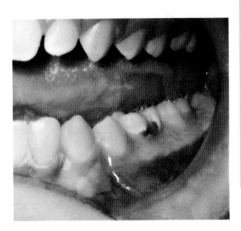

Figure 6.3 Cervical caries. Source: Reproduced by kind permission of Alan Hall.

The problems and consequences are as follows.

- sucking sweets, such as mints and toffees, leads to cervical decalcification.
- eating hard, sticky or crunchy foods damages brackets, clasps and archwires.
- fresh fruit juice and smoothies, some isotonic energy drinks, and diet and 'cola'-type drinks are acidic, attacking the enamel on the tooth surface (Figure 6.2). The result is that the tooth surface becomes glass-like, especially if the drink is swished around the teeth. Erosion of the incisal edges may lead to sensitivity (drinking straight from a can make this worse). Acid will also attack the plaque trap areas around brackets and wires.
- chewing gum can get stuck around wires and brackets.
- mints sucked slowly are often held in the buccal sulcus. They can have a high sugar content that is leached into the saliva and into the plaque, which turns to acid, leading to cervical caries (Figure 6.3).

Figures 6.4–6.8 are not the images of their teeth that patients are expecting, so show them photographs of the damage and ask them 'Is it worth the risk'?

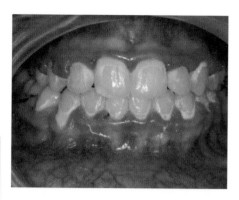

Figure 6.4 Decalcification of teeth after debanding. Source: Reproduced by kind permission of Jonathan Sandler.

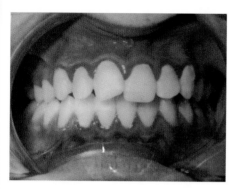

Figure 6.5 Effect of plaque on teeth. Source: Reproduced by kind permission of Jonathan Sandler.

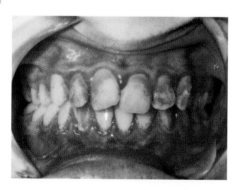

Figure 6.6 Disclosing tablets showing plaque. Source: Reproduced by kind permission of Alan Hall.

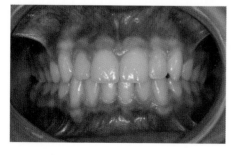

Figure 6.7 Possibly the best oral hygiene. Source: Reproduced by kind permission of Jonathan Sandler.

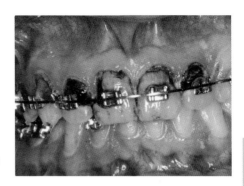

Figure 6.8 Possibly the worst oral hygiene. Source: Reproduced by kind permission of Jonathan Sandler.

WAYS PATIENTS CAN HELP THEMSELVES TO PREVENT PROBLEMS

Toothbrushes and brushing

- it does not really matter whether patients use a manual or an electric brush; it is what they do with it while it is in their mouths that counts. Some electric brushes have small heads especially designed for orthodontic use.
- patients need to have a routine, a sequence of brushing, so that every part of the mouth gets cleaned and nothing gets overlooked.
- they also need to know for how long to brush and may use a timer if that helps.
- patients should not use the same toothbrush until it is almost bald – change it regularly!
- it is advisable to clean thoroughly after breakfast and also before bedtime so that the mouth is clean overnight. Some patients use a fluoride mouth rinse.

If it is not possible to use a toothbrush when out or at school or college, then during the lunch break a vigorous rinse with water to dislodge the worst of the debris is better than nothing. However, a travel toothbrush is better. It can be washed and dried out overnight, out of its protective cover (Figure 6.9).

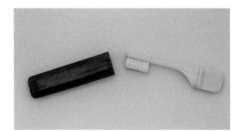

Figure 6.9 Travel toothbrush. Source: Reproduced by kind permission of Ortho-Care (UK) Ltd.

Toothpaste

It is advisable for patients to use toothpaste which contains fluoride. Some patients like to use whitening toothpaste. For those patients who don't like mint flavouring, there are some alternatives available.

ORAL HYGIENE

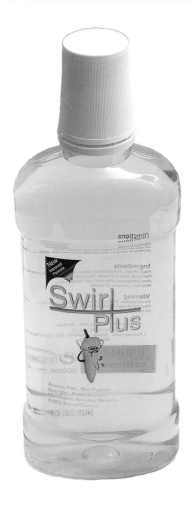

Figure 6.10 Swirl Plus fluoride mouth rinse. Source: Reproduced by kind permission of Ortho-Care (UK) Ltd.

Fluoride mouth rinse

During and after treatment a fluoride mouth rinse is recommended (Figure 6.10).

Interdental brushes

Food debris from biscuits and crisps can be soft and become easily trapped around the brackets and wires of fixed appliances or around the gingival margins of removable appliances, where it adds to the build-up of plaque. It is important that patients use interdental brushes (Figure 6.11).

Floss

Floss is not easy for younger patients to use. Getting it wound around the fingers and inserting it over and under archwires takes manual dexterity and is a learned skill and is very time-consuming.

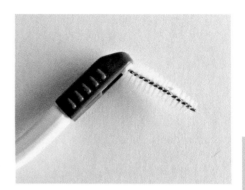

Figure 6.11 Interdental brush. Source: Reproduced by kind permission of Ortho-Care (UK) Ltd.

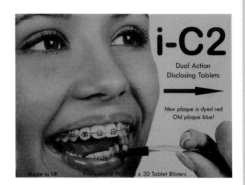

Figure 6.12 Disclosing tablets. Source: Reproduced by kind permission of Ortho-Care (UK) Ltd.

ORAL HYGIENE

Some floss is now flavoured, which is popular with patients, and some have a fluoride coating, which is popular with clinicians.

Disclosing tablets

Patients are encouraged to check that their standard of cleaning is up to scratch by using a disclosing tablet about once a week. This can be demonstrated to them at the chairside and then after that they can do it for themselves at home. Fixed appliances especially are full of little plaque traps and **must** be cleaned effectively.

After a routine brushing the patient either chews a tablet or rinses with disclosing solution for a minute. They then spit out any that is left in their mouth and look in the mirror. The plaque that is left on the teeth will be stained. The patient needs to then go back and clean their teeth again, this time being aware of the areas they are missing.

Disclosing tablets and solutions are made from vegetable dye. They are usually coloured red or blue. Tablet form is the most popular and convenient. It is helpful to check that patients do not have intolerance to erythrosine, E number 127, as it is used in some tablets. It is advisable to warn patients not to use tablets just before they are going out as they may stain the lips and tongue – a blue tinge to the lips can be a bit alarming as can a bright red tongue!

There are now tablets available that disclose both new plaque and old plaque, one being stained blue, the other red. This shows the patient the areas that need a bit more attention (Figure 6.12).

Tooth mousse

At the completion of fixed appliance treatment many clinicians encourage their patients to use tooth mousse, a water-based, sugar-free, topical cream. Tooth mousse contains calcium and phosphate but not fluoride.

Tooth mousse helps to:

- reduce sensitivity
- neutralise pH values in the saliva
- restore lost minerals
- strengthen dentine and enamel.

Fluoride toothpaste containing increased amounts of fluoride (as sodium fluoride) up to 5000 ppm (parts per million) is now available.

Both fluoride toothpaste and tooth mousse will help to reverse the effects of decalcification and to remineralise teeth.

Dietary advice

Rather than focus on what the patient cannot have, try to be positive and tell them what they can have and when is the best time to have it (Figures 6.13 and 6.14).

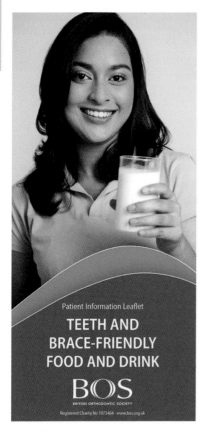

Figure 6.13 Food and drink leaflet. Source: Reproduced by kind permission of British Orthodontic Society.

ORAL HYGIENE

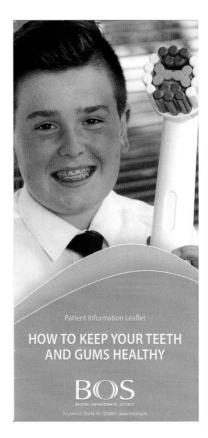

Figure 6.14 'How to keep your teeth and gums healthy' leaflet. Source: Reproduced by kind permission of British Orthodontic Society.

- chocolate is acceptable if it is broken into very small pieces and is not eaten straight from the fridge. It is best eaten with a meal that is then followed by tooth brushing.
- raw carrots, apples, and crusty bread can also be cut into tiny bite-sized mouthfuls rather than trying to bite into them.
- diluted fruit juice can be enjoyed once a day with breakfast.

Banning all the foods they like encourages patients to break the rules, so

- a little leeway helps the feel-good factor
- which helps the compliance
- which fuels the motivation
- which moves the brush!

GETTING THE MESSAGE ACROSS

Patients and their parents are always given oral hygiene leaflets, advice and instruction at each phase of their treatment (Figure 6.15). Most patients comply with the rules and they fully appreciate that it will only be for a relatively short length of time and that it will be

Why Bother to Look After Your Teeth?

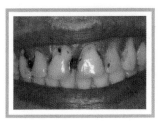

When they can look like this with no effort at all!

Figure 6.15 'Why bother to look after your teeth' leaflet.
Source: Reproduced by kind permission of Ortho-Care (UK) Ltd.

in their own best interests in the long term. Patients understand that there is no point having lovely straight teeth if the overall effect is marred by:

- enamel that is marked
- cavities, especially in the front teeth
- gum recession
- decalcification
- erosion.

When the warnings are not heard

Patients who are not keeping their mouths healthy are warned that orthodontic treatment will be terminated early if oral hygiene is falling below the expected standard. This is not a hollow threat; in extreme cases it does happen and appliances are removed before treatment has been completed.

Sometimes, patients who do not heed warnings and are facing the termination of treatment:

- ask to be given another chance
- are sorry when they realise that the appliances are being removed
- may have resigned themselves to living with irregular teeth
- often promise to try harder, in which case treatment is continued with a view to debanding as soon as possible.

The long -term damage to dental health caused by poor oral hygiene outweighs the benefits of orthodontic treatment.

Poor oral hygiene is one of the most common reasons why some patients who are eligible for, and would benefit from, orthodontic treatment do not receive it.

Nurse's role

Unlike most treatments there is no clinical procedure to follow and no instruments to prepare.

There are many ways to deliver the message:

- *the orthodontist may give the oral hygiene instruction*
- *the nurse may do it*
- *it may be a combined effort.*

If there were issues around poor cleaning before the patient was accepted for treatment and it was an area of concern which had to be improved prior to treatment being considered, you will have to be more aware and the patient will have to try extra hard to achieve the required standard.

SUPPORT

It is always useful to remember that some patients do not get the same level of home/ parental help and encouragement as others. While some patients may have a parent who buys them every brush and mouth rinse they could ever need, there are other patients who come from homes where dental care generally does not have a high priority and they get little or no support. This makes the job harder for some patients, and that makes the nurse's role harder too.

THE UNENTHUSIASTIC PATIENT

For the less enthusiastic patient, poor oral hygiene is a way of non-cooperation. It is sometimes possible to tempt this small cohort of patients by explaining that the treatment will progress much quicker if the mouth is clean. If these patients start orthodontic treatment, they, the clinician and the nurse are on an uphill struggle; they often want the appliances off as soon as possible. It is a no-win situation if this happens. You just have to try to keep them communicating with you.

THE NURSE'S ROLE

The nurse is the person who should help monitor oral hygiene and:

- *give encouragement when it is falling below standard*
- *praise when it is good.*

ORAL HYGIENE

*When a patient is doing well, **Tell them!** It is motivating just being told you are doing something positive and doing it well.*

On the other hand, if the standard is low, it is very de-motivating to hear only negative comments, even though they might be true, so try to also highlight some area that they are doing well.

Some nurses make their own oral hygiene literature and handouts. Often they compile a set of photos to show patients when they are describing what their teeth might look like if they, and the appliances, are neglected.

The oral hygiene regime that these patients are learning now will hopefully be the one that takes them all the way though life and ensures that they will have good dental health and need never lose their lovely straight teeth.

Chapter 7

Removable appliances

Teeth move as a reaction to forces applied to them.

There are two main types of orthodontic appliance:

- removable
- fixed.

Sometimes a fixed or removable appliance can have similar aims, for example:

- a fixed appliance for maxillary expansion
- a removable appliance with a central widening screw in the midline for expansion (Figures 7.1 and 7.2).

Some treatments can be completed by using removable appliances only. Removable appliances are sometimes used prior to a fixed appliance. Patients will often incorrectly refer to an active removable appliance as a 'retainer'.

At the completion of any active treatment there is a period of retention for which retainers are made. Occasionally, if treatment is with removable appliances, these can be made passive to act as retainers. Retainers are passive appliances and maintain the position of the teeth after treatment.

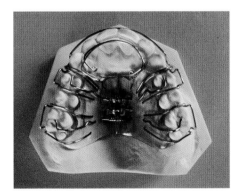

Figure 7.1 Removable appliance with expansion screw. Source: Reproduced by kind permission of Alan Hall.

Basic Guide to Orthodontic Dental Nursing, Second Edition. Fiona Grist.
© 2020 John Wiley & Sons Ltd. Published 2020 by John Wiley & Sons Ltd.

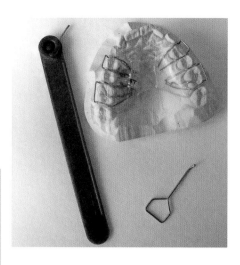

Figure 7.2 Expansion screw and choice of key types.
Source: Reproduced by kind permission of Alan Hall.

Removable appliances can move teeth using labial bows, screws, springs and elastics. Their use is not as widespread as it was, with treatment now favouring fixed appliances and aligners (see Chapter 19 on aligners).

The functional appliance is usually a removable appliance in as far as it can be taken in and out, but has different aims of treatment and is discussed in Chapter 11.

Removable appliances move teeth by tipping or tilting them, whereas fixed appliances have the ability to move teeth bodily (crown and root) without tipping. Removable appliances can be used:

- in the maxilla
- in the mandible
- both at the same time.

However, they are more often used in the upper arch. They are mostly used for the treatment of simple malocclusions or for short periods of time as part of an overall plan.

Removable appliances are most commonly used:

- as an anterior bite plane (to reduce an increased overbite)
- to move incisors over the bite (usually in the mixed dentition)
- to tip teeth labially, lingually, mesially or distally
- provide freeway space to correct an occlusal problem (disengage the occlusion)
- to widen an arch to correct a crossbite by using inbuilt expansion screws.

Like any other appliance they sometimes need to be repaired. In the case of removable appliances, this means the appliance has to be taken from the patient and sent to the laboratory. The breakage may be severe enough to make the appliance irreparable such that it is simpler for the technician to make a new one.

Removable appliances can be used in conjunction with the extraction of teeth. This provides space into which teeth can be moved in order to reduce crowding.

To be successful removable appliances must:

- be worn full time as instructed
- be worn by a keen patient
- be fitted in a clean mouth,

In addition to removable appliances with active components used to move teeth, they are also used as:

- anti-habit appliances (used to deter digit sucking)
- stimulation plates to promote eruption, where a pad of acrylic presses over an eruption site to encourage a late erupting tooth to appear
- space maintainers, worn to prevent teeth drifting
- retainers.

The components are:

- A, anchorage
- R, retention
- A, active
- B, baseplate.

The removable appliance needs to have:

- retention (to ensure the appliance is held in place), e.g. clasps/cribs
- parts to move the teeth, e.g. springs or screws
- a baseplate that fits around the teeth securely and carries all the metal components and also provides anchorage.

ADVANTAGES: WHAT THEIR BENEFITS ARE

Removable appliances:

- are simple to make by an experienced technician
- can reduce an overbite
- can tilt teeth
- are easy to wear (for children)
- need very little chairside time to fit
- facilitate oral hygiene by being removable
- are less visible.

DISADVANTAGES: WHAT THEY CANNOT ACHIEVE

Removable appliances:

- are used for simpler treatments
- cannot de-rotate teeth
- cannot move the root bodily, only tilt the position of a tooth
- can be taken out and not worn.

REMOVABLE APPLIANCES

PARTS OF A REMOVABLE APPLIANCE

Baseplate

The baseplate (Figure 7.3):

- is made of acrylic
- provides stability (anchorage) for those teeth not being moved
- carries all the active springs, screws and wires that will put force on teeth
- carries all the retention components, e.g. clasps/cribs.

Often the baseplate can include the following.

Bite plane
This can be either anterior or posterior.

Anterior
An acrylic build-up behind the upper front teeth to 'jack open' the bite so that the overbite can be reduced. Because the lower teeth bite onto plastic, it disengages the bite and allows eruption of buccal segment teeth.

Posterior
Used to include overlays over the back teeth to allow movement where there is:

- need to correct crossbites
- an increase of overbite: temporarily reducing the overbite allows upper incisor(s) to be moved 'over the bite' in Class III cases.

Anchorage

Anchorage is a point from which force is delivered. It is achieved by:

- making the acrylic baseplate fit around palatal or lingual surfaces and includes teeth other than those being actively moved
- using the baseplate together with clasps for retention of the appliance
- use of the slope of the palatal vault, e.g. when retracting upper canines and incisors (Figure 7.4).

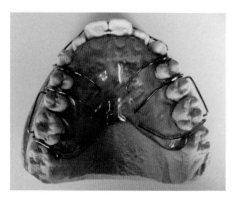

Figure 7.3 Baseplate. Source: Reproduced by kind permission of Alan Hall.

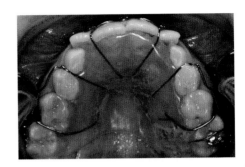

Figure 7.4 Upper removable appliance. Source: Reproduced by kind permission of Jonathan Sandler.

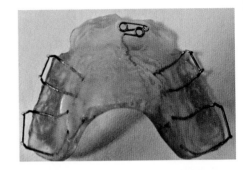

Figure 7.5 Removable appliance with Z spring. Source: Reproduced by kind permission of Alan Hall.

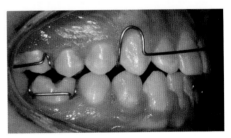

Figure 7.6 Adams clasp (crib) and a labial bow. Source: Reproduced by kind permission of Jonathan Sandler.

REMOVABLE APPLIANCES

The active components

These are the parts of the appliance that exert force. One end is embedded in the acrylic base and the other against the surface of the tooth being moved.

- springs
  - cantilever
  - Roberts retractor
  - finger
  - Z springs (Figure 7.5) and T springs
- clasps
  - Adams (Figure 7.6)
- bows
  - labial (Figure 7.6)
- screws
  - expansion
- elastics
  - can be attached from some of the metal components.

MAKING, FITTING AND ADJUSTMENT

The fitting and adjustment of removable appliances needs removable appliance pliers, acrylic burs and a handpiece for trimming. There is a huge choice of pliers and hand instruments and all clinicians have their individual preferences. As a guide, there are a number of suggested ones (as listed in Chapter 24), but they are unlikely to all be used at the same time and there may be others not mentioned.

There are now two methods of taking study models: the method detailed here using alginate impressions or by scanning the arches using an intra-oral scanner from which digital records can be made. The use of digital technology is growing apace and will in time become the method of choice, but involves significant capital outlay (for information about the digital method, see Chapter 23). Thus the traditional method will remain the norm for some while and is described in the following sections.

First appointment

For the first appointment, the nurse needs to prepare:

- *alginate, powder, liquid and liquid measure*
- *putty (vinyl polysiloxane) if preferred*
- *upper and lower impression trays*
- *bowl and spatula*
- *receiver in case of gagging reflex*
- *sheet wax*
- *heat source for wax*
- *wax knife*
- *disposable cup of mouthwash*
- *tissues*
- *laboratory sheet*
- *disinfectant solution for impressions*
- *sealable plastic bags, named and dated*
- *leaflets about removable appliances* (Figures 7.7 and 7.8).

Procedure

- *ensure that the dentist, nurse and patient wear personal protective equipment.*
- *sit patient in the upright position, for comfort when taking impressions.*
- *provide the patient with a bib, disposable cup of mouthwash, and tissues.*
- *select upper and lower trays.*
- *extend trays with ribbon wax if needed.*
- *prepare softened wax bite; this is in a horseshoe shape, two sheets of wax thick.*
- *the bite registration will then be taken.*
- *mix alginate or putty (lower impression usually taken before the upper).*
- *disinfect the alginate impressions and the wax bite.*
- *give clinician laboratory card to fill in design, etc.*

REMOVABLE APPLIANCES

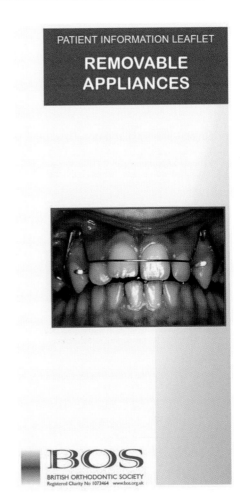

Figure 7.7 British Orthodontic Society leaflet. Source: Reproduced by kind permission of the British Orthodontic Society.

- *add the date and time of next appointment.*
- *discuss again the treatment plan and the brace with the patient.*
- *answer any questions and check the patient understands the explanatory leaflet.*
- *the disinfected impressions and wax bite then go to the technician.*

The impressions are cast to make:

- working model for the appliance
- study models.

Fitting appointment

The nurse needs to prepare:

- *clinical notes*
- *the appliance*

- *a tray* (Figure 7.9) *containing:*

  - *mirror*
  - *probe*
  - *College tweezers*

Removable Appliances

Removable appliances are specially made by a skilled technician for your mouth. They deserve to be handled with the utmost care!

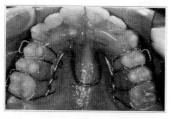

Some appliances have a deliberate split. This is not a breakage, it is the means by which tooth movement is achieved.

Fitting

When fitting the appliance into your mouth, you must take great care to ensure that the springs are placed in the correct positions. Once you are sure, the appliance can be fully seated.

Inserting your appliance

Not all appliances have springs like this, but if they do, be sure to insert the appliance correctly, or it won't work.

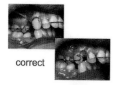

correct

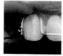

after 6 months

incorrect-no movement will occur (spring is behind tooth)

Figure 7.8 Ortho-Care leaflet. Source: Reproduced by kind permission of Ortho-Care (UK) Ltd.

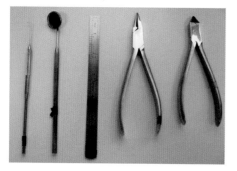

Figure 7.9 Removable appliance tray. Source: Reproduced by kind permission of Alan Hall.

- *Adams pliers* (Figure 7.10)
- *spring forming pliers*
- *ruler*
- *dividers.*

Also, there must be within reach:

- *Mauns heavy wire cutters*
- *screw key (if patient has an expansion plate)*
- *handpiece and acrylic burs*
- *Miller's articulating forceps and articulating paper*
- *sharps box for excess trimmed wire*
- *hand mirror (if you need to demonstrate to the patient)*
- *appliance box (Figure 7.11), for storage of the appliance when the patient is playing sport, a musical instrument by mouth, etc.*

Procedure

- *ensure that staff and patient wear personal protective equipment.*
- *make the patient comfortable.*
- *a straight handpiece and acrylic trimming bur are made ready.*

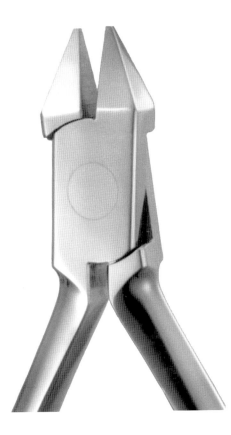

Figure 7.10 Close-up of Adams plier. Source: Reproduced by kind permission of Ortho-Care (UK) Ltd.

REMOVABLE APPLIANCES

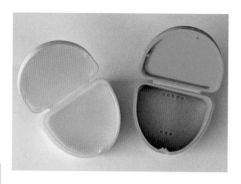

Figure 7.11 Box for storage of removable appliance when not in mouth. Source: Reproduced by kind permission of Ortho-Care (UK) Ltd.

- *articulating paper and Miller's forceps should be available.*
- *a hand mirror should be easily accessible.*
- *reassure the patient when the brace is fitted, and let the patient see themselves.*
- *encourage the patient to talk as it will feel strange and interfere with speech at first.*
- *give instructions on how to take the brace in and out and encourage the patient to try this themselves.*
- *get the patient to do this so that the parents can see this being done.*
- *discuss times it may need to be removed, and supply a protective case for these times.*
- *discuss problems which might arise from the patient playing musical instruments by mouth.*
- *give instructions on how to clean the appliance (it is helpful to advise the patient to fill the basin with water before they clean the appliance as it will 'bounce' on the surface of the water if dropped rather than fracture on impact with a hard basin).*
- *discuss the use of a mouthguard for contact sports.*
- *give lots of positive feedback on how it looks (this can worry patients).*
- *check the patient understands what to do if they are actively turning screws, etc.*
- *give the patient the turning key in a secure bag.*
- *go through the leaflet again (give them another one if it is lost).*
- *file the Medical Devices form for the appliance in the patient's notes.*

Subsequent appointments

At subsequent appointments you need the same tray set up. You also need to check with the patient that there are no problems with the brace. If there are problems and the brace is not being worn as instructed, then there will be little progress.

Some patients have problems with:

- discomfort caused by the brace (sore areas of the mouth)
- the idea of wearing it (they don't want to comply)
- social difficulties (teasing from friends, difficulty speaking in school).

You can usually tell if a brace is not being worn enough:

- it looks shiny and new
- there are few indentations in the mouth, e.g. on palatal soft tissue

- the patient has difficulty taking it in and out (not a practiced skill)
- it affects their speech (sounds like they are sucking a sweet).

If this is the case, rather than asking a closed question:

Have you been wearing your brace?

ask:

'*What do you find difficult about wearing your brace?*' or
'*When can't you wear your brace?*'

This more friendly way often gets you to the cause of the problem.

When a removable appliance has been fitted, the patient is usually instructed to wear it all the time (24 hours a day), including during eating. However, there are times when it must not be worn:

- when the patient is taking part in contact sports, such as rugby, netball or hockey
- when it is necessary to wear a protective helmet, such as for horse riding, boxing or skate-boarding
- when playing instruments by mouth
- when singing
- when swimming
- when brushing the teeth.

When someone is hit in the face with an elbow it is bad enough, but when that some-one is a patient wearing a device made of acrylic and wire it is much worse! Also, when an appliance comes out in a swimming bath it is almost impossible to find on the bottom of the pool; it is also dangerous and painful for anyone who might stand on it with bare feet.

So, when the appliance is out of the mouth it must be stored in a rigid plastic container for safety and the patient then needs to wear a mouthguard or gum shield when playing sport. It is now almost mandatory for players to wear these as some schools, colleges and clubs do not allow players on the pitch/field without one. Ideally, the retainer box should have a name and contact number in it in case it is misplaced or lost.

Another much smaller group of patients who are sometimes allowed short periods of time without the appliance are those who play musical instruments by mouth (e.g. flute, saxophone or trumpet) and vocalists who sing in choirs as part of their music syllabus.

These mouthguards/gum shields (Figures 7.12 and 7.13) can be:

- bought over the counter and moulded
- bought in approximate size
- made bespoke, by a technician.

Unlike those needed for patients wearing fixed appliances, one mouthguard will usually last the duration of the stage of treatment.

At the completion of treatment, you will need to take final impressions by either method. These are cast and trimmed as study models. If there is to be no further treatment, these may need to be boxed (Figure 7.14) and sent, with the initial set of study models, for scoring by Peer Assessment Rating (PAR, explained in detail in Chapter 3). In addition to

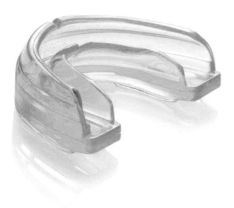

Figure 7.12 Mouthguard (single arch).
Source: Reproduced by kind permission of TOC.

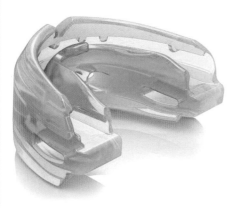

Figure 7.13 Mouthguard (both arches).
Source: Reproduced by kind permission of TOC.

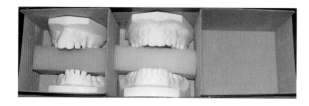

Figure 7.14 Pre- and post-treatment study models in box. Source: Reproduced by kind permission of Alan Hall.

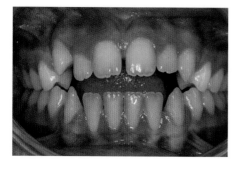

Figure 7.15 Open bite due to digit sucking. Source: Reproduced by kind permission of Jonathan Sandler.

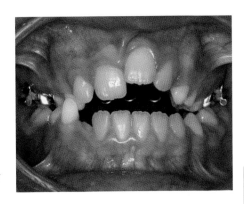

Figure 7.16 Anti-habit appliance. Source: Reproduced by kind permission of Jonathan Sandler.

pre- and post-treatment study models, these boxes can also store models taken at the end of treatment stages, Kesling set-ups and occasional work models.

If digital records are being taken, then these need to be stored securely (see Chapter 23 for storage of digital records).

Often removable appliances are used prior to fixed appliance therapy. If so, the patient may need to wear the appliance in a passive mode until the 'train tracks' are fitted.

There is another removable appliance that is passive and acts as a deterrent. This is the anti-habit appliance used to stop a patient's digit sucking habit as mentioned in Chapter 1 (Figures 7.15 and 7.16).

REMOVABLE APPLIANCES

Chapter 8

Transpalatal arches, lingual arches and quad helix

The transpalatal arch, lingual arch and quad helix are fixed appliances that are:

- fitted on teeth, most commonly on molar teeth, using bands
- usually part of standard fixed appliance therapy.

They are used to maintain space.

Sometimes when a 'd' or an 'e' is lost, their permanent successors are slow to erupt and the first permanent molars drift forwards into the space. This can happen if there is early loss due to caries for example, which would mean that the permanent successor tooth is not ready to erupt and the space would need to be held for some time.

This space may also be used:

- to correct mild anterior crowding
- to reinforce anchorage
- to hold the banded molar teeth in position while active fixed appliance treatment progresses
- to allow consolidation of the developing occlusion

After preliminary molar movements (and perhaps awaiting eruption of teeth), a transpalatal (or lingual) arch can be fitted. This can be used as a holding device and can be retained until heavy-gauge wires in the fixed appliance maintain the molar positions (Figure 8.1).

The transpalatal/lingual arch is a passive device consisting of:

- molar bands cemented onto the upper first molars
- molar bands fitted to the lower molars for a lingual arch
- a bar fitted across the palate in the upper dentition or behind the incisors in the lower
- the upper arch often has a pad of acrylic at its centre, known as a Nance button, which provides additional anchorage from the palatal vault.

The bar can be either:

- soldered to the bands in the laboratory
- fitted into a palatal or lingual tube on the band.

Basic Guide to Orthodontic Dental Nursing, Second Edition. Fiona Grist.
© 2020 John Wiley & Sons Ltd. Published 2020 by John Wiley & Sons Ltd.

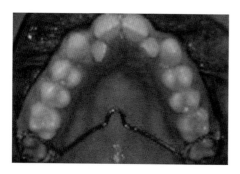

Figure 8.1 Transpalatal arch. Source: Reproduced by kind permission of Jonathan Sandler.

MAKING AND FITTING OF ARCHES

First appointment

At the first appointment the nurse will need to prepare:

- *patient's clinical notes*
- *mouth mirror*
- *dental floss*
- *posterior separating modules*
- *separating module pliers.*

Procedure

- *the nurse ensures that everyone is wearing personal protective equipment.*
- *the patient is seated comfortably in the chair.*
- *the patient is then told what is to happen and what the aim is, i.e. why this is happening and what it is going to achieve.*
- using separating module pliers, small rubber rings are placed either side of the molar around which the bands are to be fitted. (This is done several days in advance of fitting the bands as it 'springs' the teeth a tiny space apart, which makes it easier for the clinician and more comfortable for the patient when trying on the bands.)
- *the patient is then told what to expect over the next few days:*
  - *that it may be painful around the molar teeth for about 24–48 hours*
  - *what to do if a separator falls out*
  - *that if it is swallowed it will not be harmful*
  - *how to clean their teeth without dislodging the separating modules.*

Second appointment

On the second visit the nurse will need to prepare:

- *clinical notes*
- *study model box*
- *mirror, probe, College tweezers*
- *trays of appropriate molar bands*

- *bite stick*
- *floss*
- *Mershon pusher or plugger*
- *impression trays*
- *alginate, bowl, spatula (putty if preferred)*
- *receiver for gagging reflex*
- *posterior separating modules*
- *separating module pliers*
- *laboratory instruction sheet*
- *plastic bag, label and disinfectant for impression.*

Procedure

- *the nurse must ensure that everyone is wearing personal protective equipment.*
- *the patient is made comfortable in the chair.*
- the clinician will use a probe to remove the separating modules one by one. (It is important to make sure that all separators are taken out, as if accidentally left they can cause periodontal problems. For this reason, many rubber separators are radiopaque.)
- floss is used between the teeth to remove any debris.
- the correct size of band for each tooth is selected.
- these are fitted and contoured to the teeth using a Mershon pusher/plugger and bite stick, and left on the teeth.
- an alginate or putty impression is taken with the bands in position.
- the impression is removed from the mouth.
- the bands are then removed from the teeth and placed back in their correct position in the impression.
- the separating modules are replaced between the teeth either side of the first molars to maintain the space.
- *the impression is placed in disinfectant.*
- *the laboratory instructions are written, which then go to the laboratory where the impression is cast.*
- *the band sizes are recorded in the notes.*
- the palatal bar is fabricated, and the bands are soldered to it.

Fitting appointment

For the third appointment to fit the palatal or lingual arch, the nurse will need to prepare:

- *the patient's clinical notes*
- *the patient's study models*
- *work models with arches soldered to bands*
- *mirror probe and College tweezers*
- *dental floss*
- *handpiece and prophylactic paste*
- *cheek retractor*
- *cement powder and liquid*

- *pad and spatula*
- *3-in-1 syringe*
- *aspirator tube*
- *cotton wool rolls*
- *bite stick*
- *Mershon pusher/plugger*
- *Mitchell trimmer*
- *sharps box.*

Procedure

- *the nurse ensures that everyone is wearing personal protective equipment.*
- *the patient is made comfortable in the chair.*
- the separators are removed.
- floss is used to clear any debris
- the bands and arch are tried to check the fit is satisfactory.
- the cheek retractor is put in.
- the teeth are cleaned using prophylactic paste, rubber cup and contra-angled handpiece.
- all the teeth and the palatal arch are dried.
- cement is mixed and put into the inside of the molar bands which have the metal soldered to them.
- the bands and palatal/lingual arch are put into position.
- all traces of excess cement are removed.
- *the patient is given instructions on oral hygiene.*
- *the patient is given an explanatory leaflet outlining dietary restrictions, etc.*
- *the Medical Devices form from the laboratory is filed in the patient's notes.*
- *there needs to be the appropriate tray of instruments for these procedures available when required.*
- palatal and lingual arches are kept in position in the mouth until the clinician decides that they are no longer needed.
- when they need to be removed, the molar bands are lifted off and then re-cemented without the attached arch, if the treatment is to be continued.

REMOVAL OF ARCHES

The nurse will need to prepare:

- *patient's clinical notes*
- *mirror, probe and College tweezers*
- *posterior band removing pliers*
- *band slitting pliers*
- *Mitchell trimmer*
- *3-in-1 syringe*

- *handpiece, rubber cup and prophylactic paste*
- *aspirator tubes*
- *sharps box*
- *patient's model box.*

Procedure

- *the nurse needs to ensure that everyone is wearing personal protective equipment.*
- *the patient is made comfortable in the chair.*
- the clinician then uses posterior band removing pliers to gently ease the band off each tooth (use band-slitting pliers to cut the band if this is preferred).
- any cement residue is cleaned off using a Mitchell trimmer.
- the teeth are cleaned using a handpiece, rubber cup and prophy paste.
- *discarded arch and bands are disposed of in the sharps box.*

QUAD HELIX

A quad helix (Figure 8.2) has some similarities with a palatal arch. The main difference is that it is an active device used to expand the width of the upper dental arch.

It derives its name from:

- *quad*, meaning four
- *helix*, meaning circle.

Instead of having one heavy-gauge wire loop in the palate, there is a continuous length of wire into which are bent four circles that make the wire very springy. It is an appliance that is fixed to the teeth using molar bands.

In the laboratory the device is attached to molar bands which have been selected and tried in by the clinician. Following this, a work model is cast with the molar bands placed on it. The technician then fabricates the quad helix wire and solders it to the molar bands on their palatal side. (Palatal tubes for a removable quad helix can alternatively be used.)

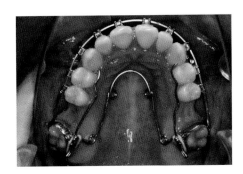

Figure 8.2 Quad helix cemented in place. Source: Reproduced by kind permission of Jonathan Sandler.

This is then cemented in following the same process as for a palatal arch but is activated by expanding the quad helix beforehand. The active spring then exerts pressure laterally and widens the arch transversely.

First appointment

For the first appointment, the nurse needs to prepare:

- *patient's clinical notes*
- *patient's model box*
- *mirror probe and College tweezers*
- *posterior separating modules*
- *separating module insertion pliers.*

Procedure

- *the nurse ensures that the dentist, nurse and patient wear personal protective equipment.*
- *the patient is made comfortable in the chair.*
- separating modules are loaded on to the pliers.
- one is placed each side (i.e. mesially and distally) to each molar tooth which is to have a band fitted onto it.
- *the patient is given an instruction leaflet.*
- *the patient is advised on:*
  - *what to do when cleaning near the separating rings, i.e. brush, not floss*
  - *what to do if the ring comes out as there is no need to panic*
  - *what foods to avoid, e.g. a very sticky or chewy diet*
  - *what to do if there is any discomfort (just take a mild analgesic).*

Some patients get very worried if they think they have swallowed a separating ring. Reassure them that if they have done, it will not do them any harm.

Second appointment

For the second appointment, the nurse needs to prepare:

- *patient's clinical notes*
- *the patient's model box*
- *contra-angled handpiece, rubber cup and prophy paste*
- *3-in-1 syringe*
- *aspirator tip*
- *trays of appropriate molar bands*
- *Mershon pusher/plugger*
- *bite stick*
- *upper impression tray*
- *alginate, bowl and spatula (putty if preferred)*
- *bowl in case of gagging reflex*

- *tissues and mouthwash*
- *solution to disinfect the impressions*
- *laboratory instruction sheet.*

Procedure

- *the nurse needs to ensure that the dentist, nurse and patient are wearing personal protective equipment.*
- *the patient is seated comfortably in the chair.*
- the separating rings are removed.
- floss is used to remove any debris.
- the bands are selected and fitted and contoured by using the Mershon pusher and bite stick.
- the impression is taken with the bands in place.
- the impression is removed and the bands placed in the correct position in the impression.
- *the impression is disinfected, labelled and bagged.*
- the laboratory sheet is written and and is sent with the impression to the technician.
- the separating rings are replaced.

Fitting appointment

At the next visit, the nurse needs to prepare:

- *the patient's model box*
- *the patient's work from the laboratory*
- *cement, powder and liquid, pad and spatula*
- *contra-angled handpiece, prophylactic paste and rubber cup*
- *3-in-1 syringe*
- *aspirator*
- *cotton wool rolls.*

Procedure

- *ensure that the patient, clinician and nurse are wearing personal protective equipment.*
- *the patient is made comfortable in the chair.*
- *the patient's models and appliance are ready.*
- *the patient's Medical Devices form is placed in the notes.*
- the separating modules are removed.
- the teeth are cleaned with handpiece, rubber cup and paste.
- the quad helix is tried in to check that it is satisfactory.
- teeth and quad helix are dried.
- *cement is mixed and used to cover the inside of the bands.*
- the quad helix is seated.
- the patient is made to bite on damp cotton wool rolls, applying pressure until cement begins to set.
- any excess cement is removed.

- *the patient is given instruction on diet, oral hygiene, etc.*
- *the patient is given the information leaflet.*

The quad helix may need a number of adjustments to achieve the upper arch expansion before this stage is completed.

REMOVAL OF QUAD HELIX

This procedure is similar to that used when taking out transpalatal or lingual arches:

- using posterior band removing pliers or band slitters the bands are eased off the teeth
- the residual cement is cleaned off
- the molar bands are replaced by either:
  - re-cementing new bands, or
  - cutting the quad helix off the original bands and re-cementing those.

NB If used bands are re-cemented, the bands must be smoothed and polished to make sure that they are not rough to the tongue.

Quad helix expansion is a preliminary phase prior to full fixed appliance therapy.

Chapter 9

Rapid maxillary expansion

When the maxilla and the mandible do not 'match' together, it can cause a transverse malocclusion. This occlusal problem is a discrepancy between a narrow or V-shaped upper dental arch form and a U-shaped lower arch. This means that the upper teeth bite inside the lower teeth on both sides (bilateral crossbites).

In order to correct the bite, the upper jaw needs to be expanded. Rapid maxillary expansion (RME) devices are cemented onto the buccal segment teeth (Figure 9.1). The appliance works by rapidly expanding the palate, the bone of which is divided in two halves by a midline suture. The appliance is cemented to teeth on each side and these are joined together by an expansion screw. The space between the two halves is initially small but every time the screw is turned this space gets wider (Figure 9.2). This appliance can be used on patients in late mixed or second dentition up to about 15 years of age.

This has similarities to distraction osteogenesis (where the bone is surgically cut prior to expansion). The gap between the two sections of bone (in the case of the palate, the midline) must fill in and consolidate with new bone.

By turning the midline palatal screw a quarter circle twice daily, the upper arch widens. Patients often feel slight discomfort in the palate. Depending on the manufacturer's instructions, the number of turns might be 40, two quarter circle turns a day for 20 days.

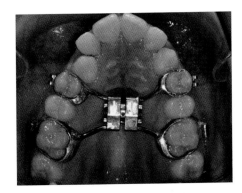

Figure 9.1 Fitting the RME. Source: Reproduced by kind permission of Jonathan Sandler.

Basic Guide to Orthodontic Dental Nursing, Second Edition. Fiona Grist.
© 2020 John Wiley & Sons Ltd. Published 2020 by John Wiley & Sons Ltd.

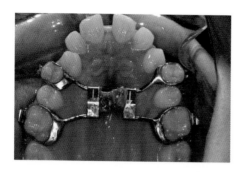

Figure 9.2 RME three weeks later. Source: Reproduced by kind permission of Jonathan Sandler.

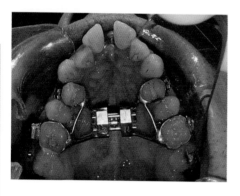

Figure 9.3 RME appliance in situ post treatment. Source: Reproduced by kind permission of Daljit Gill.

This is followed by a passive period of 2–3 months to allow consolidation of the bone in the palate. During this time the device is left in the mouth (Figure 9.3). It is good practice to fill in the screw with composite once the expansion achieved is adequate as this prevents the screw inadvertently unwinding, which could result in relapse (Figure 9.2).

When it is removed impressions are taken and a Hawley-type retainer made to maintain the position achieved. This must be fitted as soon as possible to prevent relapse of the expansion.

RME devices can be attached to the molar teeth using acrylic or molar and premolar bands. Unlike removable expansion appliances, they cannot be removed by the patient.

TAKING IMPRESSIONS

At the first appointment, the nurse needs to prepare:

- *the patient's clinical notes*
- *radiographs*
- *upper and lower impression trays*
- *alginate, bowl and spatula*
- *wax or material for bite registration*
- *wax knife*
- *method of softening wax, e.g. blowtorch, flame, hot water*

RAPID MAXILLARY EXPANSION

- *bowl for gagging reflex*
- *tissues and mouthwash*
- *solution to disinfect impressions and bite*
- *laboratory worksheets*
- *plastic bags*
- *camera (if necessary, then also lip retractors).*

Procedure

- *ensure that the patient and staff are wearing personal protective equipment.*
- *seat the patient comfortably in the chair.*
- *choose the impression tray sizes carefully.*
- *use beading wax to extend the tray if necessary.*
- record wax bite.
- *mix lower then upper alginate impressions (putty impressions if preferred).*
- *provide the patient with mouthwash and tissues.*
- *soak impressions in disinfectant tank.*
- *put impressions and bite into plastic bag with name of patient.*
- *prepare instruction sheet to go with the impressions to the laboratory.*
- *check that the patient and technician have details of the date and time of next appointment.*

Before the appliance is fitted, the patient and the person who will be turning the screw for them must have clear instructions and a demonstration of how the screw on the appliance works. This is done as a 'dry run' on the appliance before cementing it into the mouth. Several practice runs must be made to make sure this is understood and works correctly.

FITTING THE APPLIANCE

The nurse needs to prepare:

- *the patient's notes*
- *model box*
- *camera (if photos are required)*
- *cheek/lip retractors*
- *photographic mirrors*
- *appliance*
- *key to turn the expansion screw (see note below)*
- *mouth mirror*
- *probe*
- *college tweezers*
- *cement, pad and spatula*
- *Ward's carver*

- *Mitchell trimmer*
- *3-in-1 tips*
- *cotton wool rolls*
- *aspirator/saliva ejector*
- *plastic bag or box for key*
- *hand mirror*
- *leaflet.*

Procedure

- *ensure that the patient and staff are wearing appropriate protection.*
- *seat the patient comfortably in the chair.*
- allow the appliance to be tried in and the method of turning the screw explained and demonstrated until everyone is fully confident the explanation is understood.
- keep the teeth dry using 3-in-1, suction and cotton wool rolls.
- *dry the fitting surfaces of the appliance.*
- *mix the cement and fill all the fitting surfaces of the appliance.*
- *on cementing, supply two damp cotton rolls for the patient to bite on.*
- clear off excess cement gingivally with Mitchell trimmer.
- *provide the patient with mouthwash and tissues.*
- *show the patient the appliance in the mouth using the hand mirror.*
- take intra-oral and extra-oral photos (if required).
- *reassure the patient that, although it feels unfamiliar, they will soon get used to it.*
- *advise them that there is going to be a large gap opening up between the central incisors as the expansion progresses.*
- *provide a leaflet to the patient and their accompanying person.*
- *give them the key used to turn the screw (ask the accompanying person to check that they can see the screw hole and fit the key into it while the patient lies flat, as this is how they will need to do it at home) (Figure 9.4).*
- *file the Medical Devices form in the patient's notes.*
- *the patient is asked to keep a diary of their progress.*
- *check that there is an appointment arranged in 3 weeks' time.*

NB The key should either be long handled or, if short, have a length of floss attached to it so that if it is accidentally dropped while trying to turn the screw, it can be retrieved, as it could be inadvertently swallowed or inhaled.

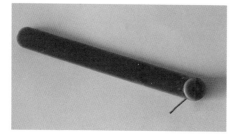

Figure 9.4 Safety swivel key for turning the screw.
Source: Reproduced by kind permission of Alan Hall.

RAPID MAXILLARY EXPANSION

WHEN SCREW TURNING HAS BEEN COMPLETED

At the next appointment, the nurse needs to prepare:

- *mirror*
- *probe*
- *college tweezers*
- *ruler*
- *dividers.*

Procedure

- *ensure the dentist, patient and nurse are wearing personal protective equipment.*
- *seat the patient comfortably in the chair.*
- check that the correct number of turns has been completed and that the screw has not been adjusted beyond that number.
- make sure that the device is still secure, that expansion has occurred and a marked upper diastema between the central incisors has appeared (Figure 9.5).
- some clinicians like to take more photographs at this point.
- *a further appointment is made for 2–3 months ahead to remove the RME and make and fit a retainer.*

WHEN THE PALATE HAS CONSOLIDATED

The nurse needs to prepare:

- *the patient's notes*
- *the patient's model box*
- *laboratory sheets*
- *bowl in case of gagging reflex*
- *plastic bag*
- *alginate, bowl and spatula*
- *impression trays*
- *wax or registration material.*

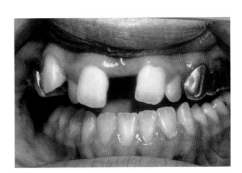

Figure 9.5 Diastema after RME appliance treatment.
Source: Reproduced by kind permission of Alan Hall.

- *method of softening wax, e.g. blowtorch, flame, hot water*
- *impression disinfection solution*
- *mirror*
- *probe*
- *Mitchell trimmer*
- *hand mirror*
- *posterior band removing pliers.*

Procedure

- *ensure that the patient and staff are wearing appropriate protection.*
- *make sure that the patient is seated comfortably.*
- remove the RME and discard in appropriate waste.
- remove any residual cement from the teeth.
- take upper and lower alginate impressions.
- record bite.
- *disinfect and bag impressions.*

Instructions are given to the technician to:

- cast study models (needed to record the end of this stage of treatment)
- cast a work model to make a passive Hawley-type retainer to maintain the expansion achieved (it is essential that this retainer is fitted the same, or the next, day as the maxillary arch expansion will begin to relapse very quickly).

FITTING THE RETAINER

The nurse will need to prepare:

- *the patient's clinical notes*
- *the patient's model box*
- *mirror, probe and College tweezers*
- *Hawley retainer appliance*
- *Adams pliers*
- *instruction leaflet*
- *straight handpiece*
- *acrylic burs*
- *retainer case.*

Procedure

The nurse should ensure that:

- *dentist, patient and nurse are wearing personal protective equipment*
- *the patient is sitting comfortably.*

RAPID MAXILLARY EXPANSION

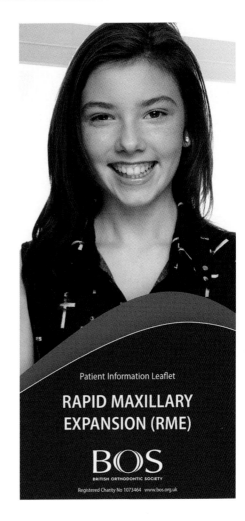

Figure 9.6 British Orthodontic Society leaflet. Source: Reproduced by kind permission of British Orthodontic Society.

The orthodontist will make sure the appliance:

- fits comfortably and is secure (adjust if necessary)
- the patient is shown how to take it in and out of the mouth (using hand mirror).

The nurse will:

- *give instructions on how to clean it (back up by giving a leaflet)*
- *advise it is to be worn, day and night, removed only for cleaning*
- *supply a retainer case*
- *name and date work and study models and put into model box*
- *file the Medical Devices form for the appliance in the patient's notes.*

The timing of the next appointment will depend on whether it is to check the retainer or to proceed direct to the next stage of treatment.

Chapter 10

Headgear

Of all the appliances, this is the one patients like least. Headgear is also known as extra-oral traction (EOT). It uses positive directional force and the anchorage is from the back of the head or neck.

To get the patient to wear it as instructed for the correct amount of time means that they need to be well motivated and compliant. It is the only appliance that is worn which has a very visible component because it is worn outside the mouth. As it is so visible, many patients are willing to wear it while they are at home but are reluctant to wear it to school or on social occasions.

The design of the head cap has now been greatly improved and efforts have been made to make it more patient friendly (Figure 10.1). They now come in a range of materials, but this has not changed the general attitude.

It can be worn in conjunction with both:

- removable appliances
- fixed appliances.

The time scale for wear varies and may be:

- full time
- 14 hours a day
- just overnight when asleep (extra-oral anchorage).

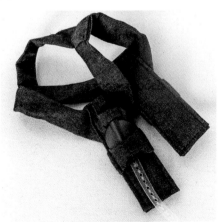

Figure 10.1 Head cap. Source: Reproduced by kind permission of Alan Hall.

Basic Guide to Orthodontic Dental Nursing, Second Edition. Fiona Grist.
© 2020 John Wiley & Sons Ltd. Published 2020 by John Wiley & Sons Ltd.

It can be used:

- to reinforce anchorage (to prevent the upper molars coming forward)
- to retract the upper buccal segments (to make enough room anteriorly).

What the headgear comprises

For conventional headgear there are several different types of head cap and cervical strap available, made from plastic or fabric, with a metal facebow. Head caps can have a backward and upward pull. Cervical (neck) straps rest on the back of the neck and have a backward but also a downward pull.

Apart from what is normally thought of as headgear, there is also a system called reverse pull headgear or protraction headgear. This system aims to advance the maxillary teeth rather than move them backwards and is used in Class III cases. It requires the use of a face frame for anchorage.

The facebow

A strong wire component that connects the intra-oral appliance to the extra-oral device.

HOW THE HEADGEAR IS ASSEMBLED

- the appliance (if removable) is fitted in the mouth.
- the inner bow of the facebow is inserted into the buccal tubes on the appliance in the mouth.
- the preformed head cap is fitted over the head.
- attached at the side of the cap in front of the ears are attachments for two sprung C modules which fit onto the sides of the head cap (Figure 10.2).
- these modules are assembled (Figure 10.3).

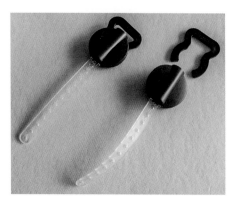

Figure 10.2 Modules. Source: Reproduced by kind permission of Alan Hall.

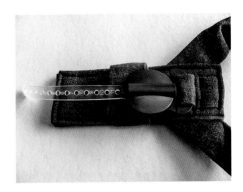

Figure 10.3 Modules fitted to head cap.
Source: Reproduced by kind permission of Alan Hall.

- the straps which are attached to them have a series of holes.
- the outer bow of the facebow terminates in hooks to which are fitted the module straps.
- the same level of hole must be used on each side of the head to maintain equal forces.
- the headgear and facebow are checked for patient comfort and correct position.

In recent years there has been great concern regarding safety when wearing these devices. These now have safety features that make them less likely to become dislodged and cause an injury to the face, and more particularly the eyes.

Clinicians strongly advise that a safety or Masel strap should always be worn, particularly when the patient is involved in close contact with other people. This is attached on one external hook and passed around the back of the neck and attached on the other one. This makes it harder to dislodge and prevents it springing back if the bow is accidentally dislodged. Modules also have safety features so that they spring apart if suddenly pulled too hard (if it were to be done accidentally).

The facebows have features on the inner bow that help prevent the bow being accidentally pulled out from the buccal tube of a fixed appliance, and have rounded ends to minimise the risk of a penetrating injury if the facebow is dislodged.

FITTING HEADGEAR

When the patient is having headgear fitted, the nurse needs to prepare:

- *the patient's clinical notes*
- *the patient's model box*
- *if a removable appliance is being used, ensure it is ready in the surgery*
- *mouth mirror*
- *Mauns heavy-duty cutters*
- *Adams pliers*
- *spring-forming pliers*
- *ruler*
- *disposable wire markers*

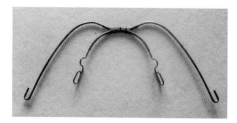

Figure 10.4 Facebow with safety locking device. Source: Reproduced by kind permission of Alan Hall.

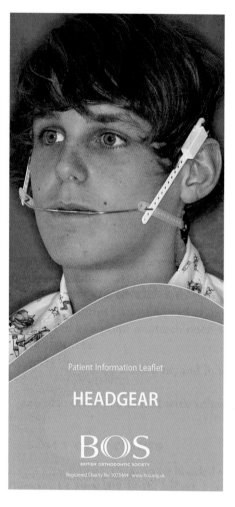

Figure 10.5 Headgear leaflet. Source: Reproduced by kind permission of British Orthodontic Society.

- *sharps box for excess cut off wire*
- *facebow (Figure 10.4) with safety locking device*
- *the C modules (these contain coil springs for force application)*
- *a hand mirror*
- *patient information and instruction leaflet (Figure 10.5).*

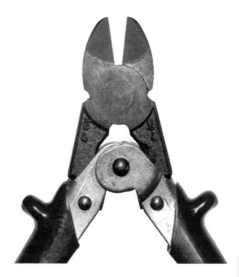

Figure 10.6 Mauns heavy-duty wire cutters. Source: Reproduced by kind permission of Ortho-Care (UK) Ltd.

Fitting the ready-made cap

- the patient is asked to choose the colour they would like.
- it is important to ensure that the skin around the ears is not rubbed.
- the correct size of facebow is selected (this should be a safety one).
- a pair of Adams pliers is used to adjust this wire.

The clinician will check that the bow fits passively into the upper first molar tubes of either the fixed or removable appliance. If the outer bow needs to be shortened, Mauns heavy-duty cutters (Figure 10.6) are used. Disposable wire markers can be used to mark the wire where it has to be cut and adjusted.

Ensure that the modules have a sufficient amount of pull. They have coil springs inside the module which applies continuous force. This can be assessed using a strain gauge. Check that when these are tugged (e.g. if done accidentally), they would spontaneously release.

CHAIRSIDE FITTING PROCEDURE

With the chosen head cap to hand, the nurse should assist the clinician.

- *ensure that the patient and staff wear personal protection.*
- *ensure that the patient is sitting comfortably.*
- if being fitted to a fixed appliance, a facebow is fitted into the upper first molar buccal tubes.
- the bow must be adjusted so that it is well clear of the upper front teeth and does not interfere with the components of the fixed appliance near the buccal tubes.
- *show the patient how to put on the head cap.*

- *demonstrate how the head cap is connected to the outer bow via the modules on the head cap.*
- *select a safety or Masel strap which fits over one end of the outer bow, around the back of the head and over the other end. This is an extra precaution. Show the patient how this is taken on and off and when it should be used.*
- *let the patient practice fitting the head cap and strapping themselves several times until they feel confident doing so.*

If the head cap is being fitted in conjunction with a removable appliance, the clinician will ensure that it fits comfortably and that the cribs have been adjusted for adequate retention. When the appliance is out of the patient's mouth, show the patient how to fit the ends of the inner bow into the tubes soldered to the upper first molar cribs (Figure 10.7). The patient can then put the combined bow and removable appliance into their mouth.

Next, show the patient how to attach the head cap. For safety reasons, with all headgear always impress on the patient:

Never put the head cap on or off with the bow attached
Never take a removable appliance out until the cap has been removed

Patients must practice and be able to assemble and remove the headgear. They must hold and stabilise the facebow with one hand whilst disconnecting the traction system with the other.

Full instructions must be given, reinforced by a written leaflet detailing:

- *how to look after the head cap*
- *for how long it must be worn each day*
- *when it should not be worn, e.g. hair washing*
- *how it is to be kept clean.*

Patients are often encouraged to fill in headgear charts or to keep a diary to record the number of hours per day that the headgear is worn.

Wearing EOT as part of appliance therapy is usually to prevent the upper first molars from coming forward. Because there is no need to distalise the teeth, merely to keep them in their normal position, only the hours of night time wear is sufficient.

For patients where there is a need to pull the upper buccal teeth distally, in order to gain space for the anterior teeth, there must be more hours of traction per day.

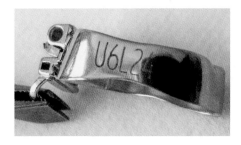

Figure 10.7 Band with tube for headgear. Source: Reproduced by kind permission of Alan Hall.

HEADGEAR

Patients who wear it in conjunction with fixed and removable appliances have routine appointments and the headgear is adjusted at the same time. The only extra equipment required is Adams pliers and Mauns heavy-duty wire cutters.

Patients who wear extra-oral systems are requested to bring these at their routine adjustment appointments during treatment together with their diary of the number of hours of wear each day.

Patients must be given a lot of encouragement. There can never be too much praise. If possible, there should be a guideline given to the patient as to how long this appliance may be needed, but a lot depends on their cooperation.

The nurse needs to prepare for all subsequent appointments for extra-oral adjustments:

- *the patient's clinical notes*
- *the patient's model box*
- *mouth mirror*
- *spring-forming pliers*
- *Adams pliers*
- *ruler*
- *Mauns heavy-duty wire cutters*
- *disposable archwire markers*
- *hand mirror*
- *sharps box.*

Chapter 11

Functional appliances

THE PROBLEM

These appliances are mainly used when correction is needed in Class II malocclusions. Their aim is to move the upper front teeth posteriorly and the lower teeth anteriorly whilst at the same time encouraging forward development of the mandible. This can reduce a significantly increased overjet (horizontal distance between the upper and lower incisor teeth) and correct a Class II molar relation to Class I.

When a patient comes into the surgery concerned that their upper teeth appear to 'stick out', they may also have:

- an underdeveloped mandible (and also a receding chin)
- a lower lip that curls under the upper teeth, often becoming trapped behind them.

This makes the upper incisors seem to protrude even further.

A clinical assessment often shows that the front teeth are not positioned too far forward in relation to the upper face. The problem is that the mandible has not grown sufficiently and is shorter than the maxilla.

The clinician may therefore decide that therapy with functional appliances is needed. These are designed to harness the power of the mandible and facial muscles to correct the occlusal relationship between the upper and lower arches. They hold the 'postured' mandible forward. This therapy is most effective in a growing patient and can be used in the later mixed dentition through puberty, when there is a growth spurt.

In very severe cases of jaw length discrepancy, particularly in older patients, orthognathic treatment (an osteotomy) is a treatment option. For less severe cases and when the patient is still growing, functional appliance therapy is often the treatment of choice.

Most functional appliances (Figure 11.1) are removable and can be taken in and out for eating and cleaning. However, the success of these appliances is related to the compliance of the patient in wearing them as advised. Patients who wear them intermittently make slow progress and, if treatment is not completed, can find that any improvement can quickly relapse.

Basic Guide to Orthodontic Dental Nursing, Second Edition. Fiona Grist.
© 2020 John Wiley & Sons Ltd. Published 2020 by John Wiley & Sons Ltd.

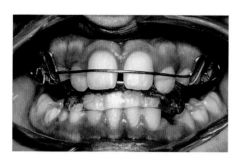

Figure 11.1 Functional appliance in the mouth. Source: Reproduced by kind permission of Alan Hall.

THE SOLUTION

The functional appliance works by movement of the teeth and alveolar bone with some forward mandibular development too.

This therapy relies on oro-facial muscles to supply the force which, transmitted through the functional appliance, produces intermaxillary traction. Before the appliance is fitted, the overjet is measured and recorded and this is done again at each follow-up appointment and at the end of treatment.

When the treatment is completed it should be possible to gradually remove the appliance and find that the mandible and occlusion remain stable in what was initially seen to be a 'postured' position.

TYPES OF FUNCTIONAL APPLIANCE

There are many types of functional appliance and because there seems to be no accepted classification, many are known by the name of the clinician who developed them. For example, the **Andresen** activator is:

- a tooth-borne appliance
- basically an upper and lower appliance fused together, where the lower one is advanced forward of the upper
- made of acrylic and wire
- successful on Class II/I cases with well-aligned arches.

The **Frankel** function regulator:

- is a soft tissue-borne appliance
- has lip and cheek bumpers
- is made of acrylic and wire
- is used in mixed and early second dentition.

The **Clark Twin Block** (Figures 11.2, 11.3, 11.4 and 11.5):

- is a tooth-borne appliance
- is made of acrylic and wire

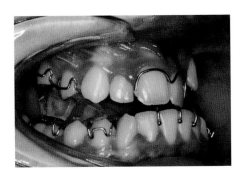

Figure 11.2 Clark Twin Block: lateral view. Source: Reproduced bykind permission of Jonathan Sandler.

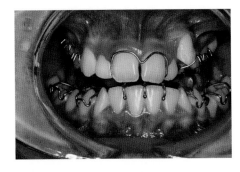

Figure 11.3 Clark Twin Block: front view. Source: Reproduced bykind permission of Jonathan Sandler.

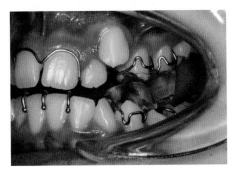

Figure 11.4 Clark Twin Block: lateral view. Source: Reproduced bykind permission of Jonathan Sandler.

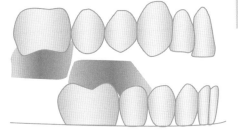

Figure 11.5 Diagram of position of blocks on appliances. Source: Reproduced by kind permission of Alan Hall.

- is an appliance in two separate parts
- is worn on the upper and lower arches
- has close-fitting baseplates which makes it well tolerated
- has angled bite blocks which posture the mandible forward and the two parts slide over one another

FUNCTIONAL APPLIANCES

- is compatible with the wearing of headgear
- is very popular with patients in the UK.

The **Harvold** appliance:

- is a tooth-borne appliance
- is made of acrylic and wire
- holds the bite well open.

The **Medium Open Activator** (MOA) (Figure 11.6):

- is a tooth-borne appliance
- is made of acrylic and wire comprising
    - upper baseplate
    - labial bow
    - cribs for retention
    - lower acrylic extension into which the lower incisors bite to posture the mandible forward
- is smaller than conventional functional appliances
- is easier to wear.

These functional appliances are all **removable** appliances.

The **Herbst functional appliance** is an appliance which is **fixed** to the teeth. The Herbst appliance (Figure 11.7):

- is sometimes used when there is poor compliance and the patient will not wear a removable appliance for sufficient hours to make it effective
- is made with upper and lower components which are connected by telescopic pistons

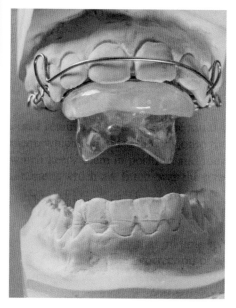

Figure 11.6 MOA showing rest for lower teeth in the postured position. Source: Reproduced by kind permission of Alan Hall.

FUNCTIONAL APPLIANCES

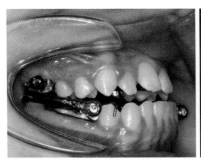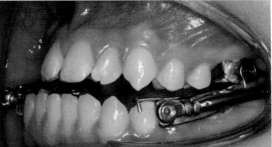

Figure 11.7 Herbst appliance. Source: Reproduced by kind permission of Jonathan Sandler.

- is well tolerated and comfortable to wear because of the easy range of vertical and some lateral movement the appliance
- ensures a higher level of success as being cemented in place means that the patient has no option but to wear it full time.

These appliances call for a high degree of compliance in a well-motivated patient. The choice of functional appliance used depends on factors in the malocclusion and the personal preference of the orthodontist.

FIRST APPOINTMENT

For the first appointment, the nurse needs to prepare:

- *the patient's clinical notes*
- *orthopantomogram (OPT) and lateral cephalometric radiographs*
- *mouth mirror*
- *ruler*
- *alginate, bowls and spatula (putty, i.e. vinyl polysiloxane, if preferred)*
- *upper and lower impression trays*
- *wax*
- *bite stick (if needed) to assist patient in making a postured bite*
- *method of softening wax*
- *supply of cold water in container to chill the wax bite*
- *mouthwash and tissues*
- *solution to disinfect impressions and bite*
- *plastic bag and gauze*
- *laboratory instruction card*
- *clinical camera*
- *lip and cheek retractors*
- *photographic mirrors*
- *next date for fitting appointment*
- *information leaflet about functional appliances for patient* (Figures 11.8 and 11.9).

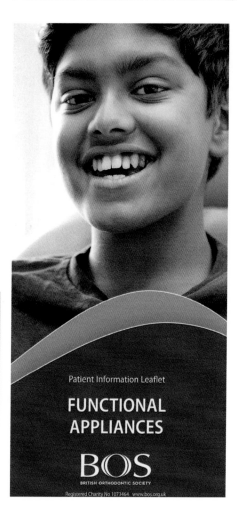

Figure 11.8 British Orthodontic Society leaflet. Source: Reproduced by kind permission of the British Orthodontic Society.

FUNCTIONAL APPLIANCES

Procedure

- *the nurse ensures the patient and staff wear personal protection.*
- *the nurse ensures the patient is comfortable.*
- intra-oral and extra-oral photographs are taken.
- a bite is taken in normal centric occlusion (as the patient bites).
- using several thicknesses of wax, another bite is taken in the postured position (with the mandible biting in a forward position).
- a supply of cold water in a suitable container is needed (the bite is removed from the mouth and cooled before trying it in again to check there has been no distortion).
- upper and lower alginate or putty impressions are taken.
- *impressions and bite are disinfected before they go off to the laboratory.*
- *the patient is instructed in how and when the appliance is to be worn.*
- *the patient is told how to clean the appliance.*

Why Functional Appliances?

Apparent prominence of the upper front teeth can be due as much to a small retruded lower jaw. Functional appliances are designed to encourage as much forward movement of the lower jaw and teeth as possible to improve the facial profile and avoid over retraction of the upper front teeth.

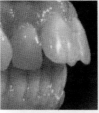 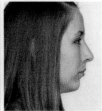

Upper front teeth too far forward?   *Lower jaw too far back?*

Functional appliances therefore give the best chance of balancing the profile with the positions of the teeth whilst producing the most pleasing appearance.

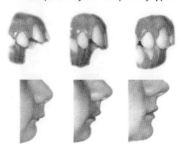

Figure 11.9 Ortho-Care leaflet. Source: Reduced by kind permission of Ortho-Care (UK) Ltd.

FUNCTIONAL APPLIANCES

- *arrangements for wearing brace are discussed if the patient plays an instrument by mouth; if patient plays contact sports, they should wear a mouthguard.*
- *laboratory design instructions and diagram, and sterilised impressions and bite are sent to the technician.*
- *the patient is given an information leaflet about the functional appliance.*

FITTING APPOINTMENT

At the fitting appointment, the nurse will need:

- *appliance to be fitted*
- *hand mirror*

- *patient's model box*
- *mouth mirror*
- *ruler*
- *Adams pliers*
- *straight handpiece and acrylic bur*
- *instruction leaflet*
- *functional appliance case*
- *hand mirror*

Chairside procedure

The nurse will then:

- *ensure that the patient and staff wear personal protection*
- *make the patient comfortable in the chair*
- *assist the clinician in fitting the appliance, ensuring that it is firm and lower teeth fit comfortably into the appliance in the forward position*
- *show the patient how to remove and insert appliance correctly*
- *record the starting overjet with the appliance out of the mouth*
- *go over the information and instruction leaflet again*
- *give the patient a functional appliance case (Figure 11.10) in which to keep the appliance when it is out of the mouth (e g. cleaning, contact sports)*
- *ask the patient and the parent if they have any questions*
- *advise the patient and parent of the amount of overjet reduction being aimed for at the conclusion of this phase of treatment*
- *explain to patient how and when it is to be worn*
- *tell patient how to clean the brace (after every meal and weekly with special cleaner, e.g. Retainer Brite)*
- *confirm arrangements for wearing brace if the patient plays instruments by mouth*
- *confirm arrangements if patient plays contact sports and wears a mouthguard*
- *advise the patient to keep a diary of times of wear.*

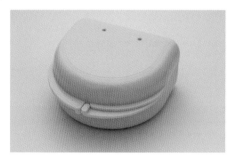

Figure 11.10 Case for functional appliance. Source: Reduced by kind permission of Ortho-Care (UK) Ltd.

SUBSEQUENT APPOINTMENTS

- the same format is followed until the measurement of the overjet has reduced to that planned for.
- the molar relationship should also be checked that this is being corrected.
- when the required measurement has been reached, further impressions will be taken to record the end of that stage of treatment.
- if the patient is then to have fixed appliance therapy, the functional appliance will be worn at nights only to hold the correction achieved until the fixed appliance is fitted. Some clinicians trim the functional appliance at this stage to help eliminate any lateral open bite which has developed.
- functional appliances cannot align irregular teeth or arches, so most patients then move into fixed appliance therapy.

When fitting the functional appliance, patients need to be given a functional appliance case. In the unlikely event of it being lost, marking the patient's name inside is helpful. This case is larger than a removable appliance or retainer case as many functional appliances are much bulkier, especially in height.

Patients receive the same instructions as those wearing removable appliances about not wearing their appliances for contact sports, swimming, any sport that needs a helmet such as horse riding or skateboarding, and when playing musical instruments by mouth. Cleaning the appliance is the same as for removable appliances and retainers.

FUNCTIONAL APPLIANCES

Chapter 12

Temporary anchorage devices and magnets

WHAT THEY ARE

Orthodontic treatment and treatment philosophies are always moving forward. The use of a temporary anchorage screw has expanded the scope of clinical work and clinicians can now create an anchorage site exactly where they need it.

Temporary anchorage devices (TADs) are also known as:

- mini screws
- mini implants.

The TAD is made of a medical-grade biocompatible titanium alloy. It is literally a screw that is inserted through the gum and into the alveolar bone.

WHAT THEY DO

In orthodontic treatment some teeth are used for anchorage, from which a force is applied to the teeth to be moved. This may be in the same dental arch or the opposing one. However, they may not always be in the right position or at the right angle to do this, but by fitting a small screw a more precise anchorage site can be achieved.

There is now an increased range of treatments available to the clinician when using fixed and immovable anchor points; these can be for diverse uses, such as correcting open bites, uprighting molars or closing spaces. Because the clinician can usually position it where it is needed, it will optimise the results and increase the range of tooth movements achievable.

Extra anchorage points are also useful when:

- the existing teeth are not suitable or insufficient
- the force might not move the teeth correctly
- the teeth required are not present (hypodontia).

The use of these devices also has advantages for patients. TADs are all intra-oral and the effectiveness of their treatment is improved.

Basic Guide to Orthodontic Dental Nursing, Second Edition. Fiona Grist.
© 2020 John Wiley & Sons Ltd. Published 2020 by John Wiley & Sons Ltd.

THE ADVANTAGES OF TADS

The advantages of mini screws are as follows:

- they are quick and easy to use
- they have a success rate of over 75%
- they can be sited where the orthodontist thinks they will be of most benefit
- they can also provide an alternative to wearing headgear
- once fitted, they can be used straight away (no consolidation period)
- it is a relatively painless procedure, needing only a local anaesthetic on insertion
- they are screwed directly into the bone
- any mild discomfort lasts only a few days
- screws can safely be left *in situ* for several months
- screws are easily and painlessly removed
- once removed, the site heals quickly
- mini screws are relatively inexpensive.

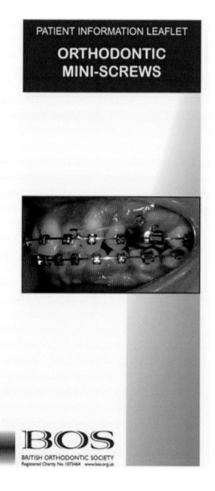

Figure 12.1 British Orthodontic Society leaflet. Source: Reproduced by kind permission of the British Orthodontic Society.

TEMPORARY ANCHORAGE DEVICES

THE DISADVANTAGES OF TADS

The disadvantages of TADs are:

- they can fail
- they can become loose
- they can break
- on insertion, they can come into contact with a root
- the site can become infected
- the start-up cost of equipment.

The added oral hygiene requirements for mini screws are basically:

- a chlorhexidine rinse for a week after insertion
- gentle manual brushing with fluoride toothpaste after meals while in place.

HOW THE DEVICE IS FITTED

When the TAD is fitted, the patient will feel some discomfort, like a pressing feeling. This passes off very quickly, but some clinicians like to apply a little topical anaesthetic to the area followed by a small local anaesthetic injection. It takes only a few minutes to insert these devices, during which time the patient feels only minimum discomfort (Figures 12.2, 12.3 and 12.4).

The patient is given patient comfort wax or medical-grade silicone to use if the screw should cause irritation by rubbing the soft issues on the inside of the mouth.

It is possible to buy a kit which supplies the contra-angled hand driver, tips, screwdriver handle, screwdriver tips and pilot drill. All attachments can be bought individually, including post heads, bracket head, contra-angled tips and screwdriver tips. All screws come prepacked in sterilisable envelopes. Separate sterilisation trays are also sold with these kits (Figure 12.5).

Because the device is basically a screw, it is inserted using a screwdriver. When the time comes to remove the device, after putting a little topical anaesthetic on the gum around the site, the screwdriver turns the screw in the other direction and gently eases it out. This procedure takes roughly the same length of time as it did to put it in. The site heals rapidly.

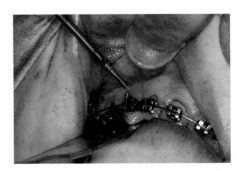

Figure 12.2 TAD being inserted. Source: Reproduced by kind permission of Steven Jones.

TEMPORARY ANCHORAGE DEVICES

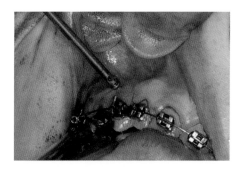

Figure 12.3 TAD fully inserted. Source: Reproduced by kind permission of Steven Jones.

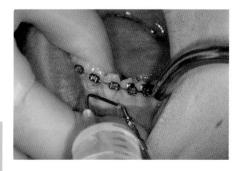

Figure 12.4 TAD being inserted. Source: Reproduced by kind permission of Jonathan Sandler.

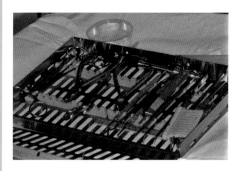

Figure 12.5 TAD tray. Source: Reproduced by kind permission of Jonathan Sandler.

The advantages outweigh the disadvantages. This is a technique that expands the scope of orthodontic treatment in a unique way; however, it is a temporary measure, not intended to be used for long periods. The procedure is user friendly, the screw easy to fit and ready to use straight away, but must be undertaken using sterile techniques.

The screw is made of titanium alloy and is available in different lengths and thicknesses depending into which part of the mouth it is to be inserted.

- the longest (10 mm) screw is for areas of thick bone:
  - the infra-zygomatic crest
  - the molar regions of the mandible
- the middle size (8 mm) screw is for facial and lingual areas of the maxilla:
  - tooth-bearing areas of the mandible

TEMPORARY ANCHORAGE DEVICES

- the smallest size (6 mm) screw is for the facial area of the maxilla:
  - tooth-bearing areas of the mandible.

The clinician selects which one is most appropriate to use and decides what is to be attached to the device, for example:

- thread elastic
- linked chain
- coil
- NiTi coil spring
- archwire.

Preparation

The nurse needs to prepare:

- *the patient's clinical notes*
- *the patient's radiographs and models*
- *mirror, probe and College tweezers*
- *small pledget of cotton wool*
- *gel for topical anaesthesia (and cartridge syringe, disposable needle and ampoule if local injection is to be given)*
- *tray set up for the procedure also taking place*
- *3-in-1 syringe*
- *fine-tipped surgical (Frazier) aspirator*
- *lip retractor*
- *cotton wool rolls*
- *a fixed appliance tray and sundries to adjust the appliance*
- *a TAD fitting tray*
- *tissues and a glass of mouthwash*
- *sharps box*
- *hand mirror*
- *instruction leaflet on oral hygiene*
- *box of relief wax or medical-grade relief silicone.*

Procedure

The nurse needs to assist the clinician at the chairside by:

- *ensuring that the patient and staff all wear personal protection*
- *seating the patient comfortably in the chair*
- *ensuring that access to the site is clear*
- *ensuring that the anchorage fitting kit is laid out ready*
- *ensuring that the method of attaching the screw to the appliance is ready to use, e.g. coil, springs or linked chain*
- *assisting with a fixed appliance adjustment in addition to fitting the temporary screw*
- *giving the patient an instruction leaflet on care of the device*
- *giving the patient oral hygiene instructions*

- *making sure that the patient understands what the signs might be if something was not right*
- *ensuring that the patient has mouthwash and patient comfort wax*
- *giving the patient the next appointment.*

When these appliances have outlived their usefulness, they can be very easily removed. The benefits of this procedure are:

- it does not necessarily require an anaesthetic
- it does not cause the patient pain
- the site heals very quickly
- it leaves no lasting damage to bone or soft tissue.

These devices are an extension of what the younger patient may expect as part of their treatment and is often a scary prospect. The nurse will pick up on this and is a good person to give reassurance and advice to both patients and parents.

Frequently asked questions

Some frequently asked questions include the following.

Will it hurt?

Reassure the patient. The screw is very small, there will be little local anaesthetic used and they should not feel anything more than a gentle pressure. Advise them that with all the pushing it might be a bit sore that evening but if it is, just take the tablet you would take if you had a headache, and it will be gone in the morning.

For how long will I have to have it?

Explain that it will be in as short as possible but it is hard to predict at the beginning, as the orthodontist cannot tell exactly how long the treatment will take but once started will be able to give the patient a better idea. It is usually no more than a few months, but emphasise that it will be taken out a soon as it has done its job.

What if the screw rubs my cheek or tongue?

Because it is new in the mouth, it may rub the tongue and soft tissues – it is strange and foreign to them. This will quickly pass, like getting used to new trainers, but if it gets sore, just use a little orthodontic wax.

How do I look after it?

For the first few days, rinse a couple of times with a chlorhexidine antibacterial mouthwash. Put your toothbrush in the solution and clean around the area gently. If you use an electric toothbrush, don't risk using it near the mini screw in case you knock it. Try to forget it is there. Don't fiddle with it!

What happens when it comes out?

Usually the screw comes out really easily and you don't need a local anaesthetic or feel anything. Within a few days the site is healed and there is nothing to see!

As the nurse, you are in an excellent position to reassure and are helped by the fact that you are giving the good news the patient and their back-up team want to hear.

The National Institute for Health and Care Excellence (NICE) has produced information on this procedure for patients. It is available from www.nice.org.uk/IPG238publicinfo.

The use of these devices will expand many treatment options in the future. This may have particular implications in areas where specific and additional anchorage is needed, such as hypodontia cases.

MAGNETS

For many years there has been research into various techniques for using magnetic force to try to copy conventional orthodontic methods for inducing movement. Magnetic force can be:

- attractive or repulsive
- is measured in grams.

There are many advantages to these treatments, including:

- ability to achieve both dental and orthopaedic change
- can decrease treatment time
- are safe
- involve less discomfort for the patient
- forces are continuous
- do not cause root resorption or caries.

Their uses are extensive and include:

- space closure
- tooth movement
- palatal expansions
- extrusion
- retraining tooth position post treatment
- guiding unerupted or impacted teeth (Figures 12.6 and 12.7).

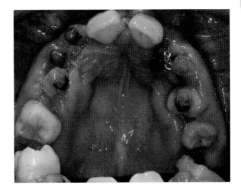

Figure 12.6 Magnets *in situ*. Source: Reproduced by kind permission of Jonathan Sandler.

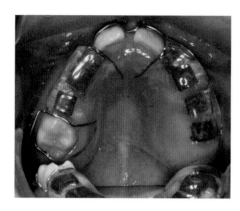

Figure 12.7 Magnets *in situ*. Source: Reproduced by kind permission of Jonathan Sandler.

Chapter 13

Fixed appliances: what they do and what is used

This chapter concentrates on what is meant by fixed appliance therapy and what the nurse needs to prepare when a fixed appliance is either fitted or adjusted in the surgery.

Fixed appliance therapy:

- moves teeth with far greater accuracy and control than removable appliances
- normally moves a number of teeth at the same time
- is more sophisticated than a removable appliance
- can move crowns and the roots of teeth bodily, not just tip them
- can be used with extraction or non-extraction treatments
- is sometimes used following removable or functional appliance treatment
- can be worn with headgear appliances (e.g. night-time to prevent first molars drifting forwards)
- is used in conjunction with multidisciplinary treatments such as orthognathic surgery and in hypodontia cases.
- cannot be taken in and out by the patient.

When patients speak of orthodontic treatment, the majority of teenagers think of fixed appliances (Figures 13.1, 13.2 and 13.3), a system they often refer to as 'train tracks'. A look at clinic lists would reveal a high proportion of 'fixed' adjustment appointments on them.

PATIENT EXPECTATION: THE POPULAR CULTURE OF TRAIN TRACKS

For most patients of typical orthodontic age, this is the appliance that they would all prefer if they had the choice. It is regarded:

- as the gold standard, 'the proper brace'
- that braces that are removable are often seen as inferior
- it is fashionable, most of their friends have it, and it gives them status.

Much discussion of their treatment goes on during school break times and experiences are exchanged.

Basic Guide to Orthodontic Dental Nursing, Second Edition. Fiona Grist.
© 2020 John Wiley & Sons Ltd. Published 2020 by John Wiley & Sons Ltd.

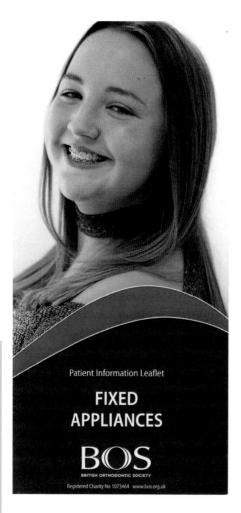

Figure 13.1 British Orthodontic Society leaflet. Source: Reproduced by kind permission of the British Orthodontic Society.

FIXED APPLIANCES

PEER PRESSURE

Most teenage patients like to be seen:

- to have the same appliances as their friends
- to be part of the crowd.

Patients have their own language when talking about fixed appliance treatment. Apart from the system being known as 'train tracks', they call:

- the appliance 'braces'
- the bands 'rings'
- the brackets 'blocks'.

By definition, it is a system that is fixed to the teeth and one which the patient is not able to remove.

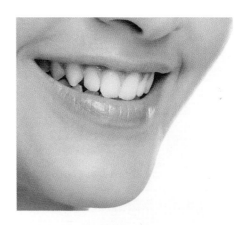

Fixed
Orthodontic
Appliances

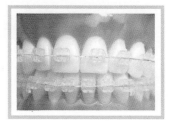

Figure 13.2 Ortho-Care leaflet. Source: Reproduced by kind permission of Ortho-Care (UK) Ltd.

STAGES OF TREATMENT IN FIXED APPLIANCE THERAPY

There are four stages in fixed appliance therapy.

- alignment: aligning irregular teeth including rotations, height differentials, etc.
- working: resolving abnormal overbites and overjets and space closure after extractions.
- finishing: torquing incisors and fine aesthetic detailing.
- retention: maintenance of the treatment results with retainers.

Fixed appliances can be fitted to the teeth by either:

- direct bonding
- indirect bonding.

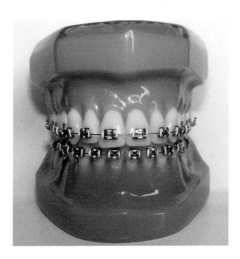

Figure 13.3 Upper and lower fixed appliances with metal brackets. Source: Reproduced by kind permission of Alan Hall.

WHAT IS USED IN FIXED APPLIANCE THERAPY?

The basic mechanics of 'train tracks' are:

- each tooth has an attachment fitted to it
- initially, a fine archwire is fitted into these attachments
- the teeth can be moved along this wire into alignment or be moved by the flexibility of the archwire itself.

In order to do this, the system uses:

- bands (on molar teeth)
- brackets
- buccal tubes (on molar teeth)
- wire.

Brackets and buccal tubes are bonded to the teeth with composite adhesive and glass ionomer cements. Molar bands are first fitted to the teeth and then cemented. These provide 'handles' on the teeth which engage the archwire.

The capability of fixed appliances is such that a finished result should include:

- a balanced occlusion (all teeth biting evenly together)
- no residual spacing
- no rotated or submerged teeth
- an acceptable gumline (the margins look even).

While removable appliances can expand arches and tip teeth, the fixed appliance is more sophisticated. It has many applications and can achieve many kinds of tooth movement:

- positional
- rotational
- extrusion and intrusion of teeth
- torquing the roots.

FIXED APPLIANCES

THE ATTACHMENTS

- bands
- brackets
- buccal tubes, buttons, eyelets and cleats.

Bands

Bands are fitted exactly around a tooth, usually on the molars, and being in the masticatory regions of the dentition provide extra strength. (In some cases, however, buccal tubes may be sufficient.)

Molar bands (Figure 13.4) are:

- usually made of stainless steel
- pre-formed and come in a large range of sizes
- used on both first and second molars
- have buccal tubes welded to accommodate both archwire and headgear (Figure 13.5)
- have size and quadrant etched onto the surface of each band for identification
- have a straight occlusal edge, the gingival edge being contoured
- stored in separate trays, for each molar and quadrant (Figure 13.6), so eight trays are for single use only (if a patient's band comes loose, it can be re-cemented but not used for another patient).

If the molar bands are to be used as part of a transpalatal or lingual arch system, the bands will be soldered to the arch. The other teeth in the arch anterior to the first molars are

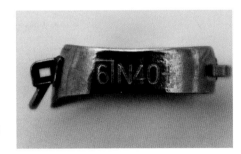

Figure 13.4 Molar band with tube. Source: Reproduced by kind permission of Alan Hall.

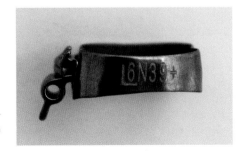

Figure 13.5 Band with additional slot on buccal tube for headgear. Source: Reproduced by kind permission of Alan Hall.

FIXED APPLIANCES

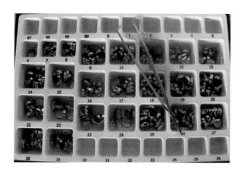

Figure 13.6 Tray of first molar bands.
Source: Reproduced by kind permission of Alan Hall.

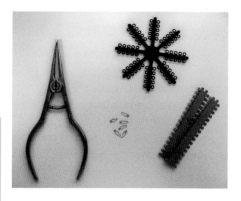

Figure 13.7 Green anterior and blue posterior separating rings, separating springs and separating pliers. Source: Reproduced by kind permission of Ortho-Care (UK) Ltd.

FIXED APPLIANCES

fitted with brackets. This allows the archwire which fits into the bracket slots to continue further back into a buccal tube which is attached to the side of the band. There are a great many variations on the size and type of buccal tubes that can be used.

Bands can:

- have a variety of auxiliaries:
  - single tubes
  - double tubes
  - triple tubes.
- have cleats welded to them, palatally or lingually
- have triple tubes if two archwires are being used and headgear can also be fitted.

Separation

Bands cannot be fitted in cases of crowding and tight contact points unless the patient has worn separating modules to create an interproximal space to allow the band to be seated comfortably and accurately. These are fitted several days prior to the band fitting to open the contact point. They are placed between the teeth using separating pliers. Springs are occasionally used, placed by pliers, especially for partially erupted teeth (Figure 13.7).

Brackets

Brackets can be made of:

- stainless steel (Figure 13.8)
  - the most commonly used in the growing patient
  - tooth friendly
  - not as hard as ceramic brackets so not likely to fracture with a direct blow (sports, etc.)
- aesthetic material (Figure 13.9)
  - tooth coloured or clear
  - not as noticeable
  - superior aesthetics
  - preferred by adults
  - often have metal insert in the archwire slot as metal slides well over metal, resulting in less friction and more efficient movement of teeth
  - slightly bulkier.

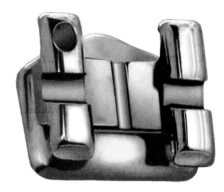

Figure 13.8 Metal bracket. Source: Reproduced by kind permission of Ortho-Care (UK) Ltd.

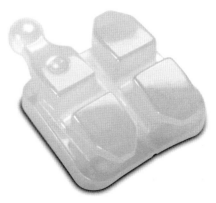

Figure 13.9 Clarity™ aesthetic bracket. Source: Reproduced with permission from 3M Unitek © 2019. All rights reserved.

FIXED APPLIANCES

Brackets can be:

- fixed to the labial and buccal surfaces of the teeth (more easily accessible for the clinician but visible)
- fixed to the lingual (palatal and tongue) surfaces of the teeth (i.e. not visible)
- be self-ligating or conventional, requiring the archwire to be held into the bracket with ligatures or O-rings.

They have a rectangular section channel (slot) in the bracket which houses the archwire. Round section wires do not fit as snugly as rectangular wires. This allows some 'play' while rectangular wires are more firmly engaged.

- brackets are almost always of the pre-adjusted design.
- the prescription dictates the levels of tip and torque (torque is the correction of inclination labio-lingually).
- these can be to different prescriptions, e.g. Roth, Andrews and MBT (McLauglin, Bennett and Trevisi).
- each tooth has its own prescribed individual bracket.
- some brackets are self-ligating with mechanics built into holding the wire.
- pre-adjusted brackets developed from the Begg technique are marketed as the Tip Edge system.

The archwire is held positively in the bracket by a metal ligature or an elastomeric. Some self-ligating brackets do not use this method:

- they have a latch built into the bracket itself, which makes it self-ligating
- the latch is opened to insert or remove the archwire using a special tool that opens and closes the latch.

Brackets can either:

- be fixed to the tooth by applying composite adhesive in the surgery
- come from the manufacturer ready pre-coated with adhesive (Figure 13.10).

   There are two techniques for doing this.

- direct bonding: fixing the individual attachments directly onto the teeth (most commonly used).
- indirect bonding: positioning them on a model, transferring them to a tray, placing the tray in mouth and curing them together through the tray.

It is crucial that the brackets are placed very accurately because if they are at the wrong height or angulation, the tooth will not subsequently align correctly.
   Therefore, brackets have the following characteristics.

- they are usually mounted on orientation cards for ease of delivery (Figures 13.11 and 13.12).
- they often have a coloured identification dot to show which way up they are and for which tooth.
- they have angles of torque as well as tip built into the wire slot.
- popular prescriptions are Roth, Andrews and MBT.

FIXED APPLIANCES

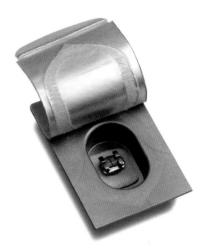

Figure 13.10 VS™ PLUS adhesive-coated appliance system, open blister. Source: Reproduced with permission of 3M Unitek © 2019. All rights reserved.

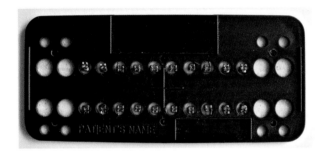

Figure 13.11 Metal brackets on orientation card. Source: Reproduced by kind permission of Ortho-Care (UK) Ltd.

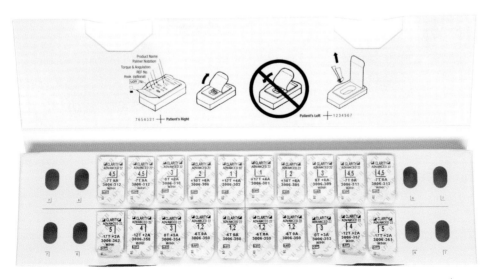

Figure 13.12 Clarity™ advanced adhesive-coated bracket system on orientation card. Source: Reproduced with permission of 3M Unitek © 2019. All rights reserved.

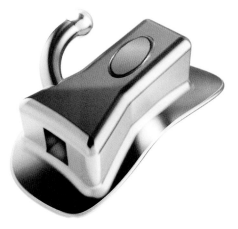

Figure 13.13 Buccal tube. Source: Reproduced by kind permission of Ortho-Care (UK) Ltd.

- canine brackets can have 'hooks' to aid elastic wear (osteotomy patients often need hooks on canines and premolars).
- they have bases that are textured for extra glue retention.
- they are contoured to the surface of the tooth.

Buccal tubes

Buccal tubes are an attachment in their own right (Figure 13.13). They are used when the fixed appliance does not need to include molar bands, All attachments are bonded.

The buccal tube can come with or without a hook. The hook is placed toward the gingival as opposed to the occlusal part of the tooth. The direction of the hook is towards the back of the mouth, i.e. the 'open' end faces distally. This hook has a function similar to a hook which forms part of a bracket or a crimpable hook that is fixed onto an archwire. It can be used as a point to attach inter- or intra-maxillary elastics.

Buccal tubes:

- can be used both instead of, and in addition to, molar bands on first and second molars
- can also come pre-coated with adhesive.

Eyelets and cleats

Extra attachments that can be bonded onto molar or other teeth to provide traction points (Figures 13.14 and 13.15).

ARCHWIRES

A wide range of archwires is available and each clinician has their own preferences. They can be on spools or in lengths to be custom made or they are pre-formed and sold in packs.

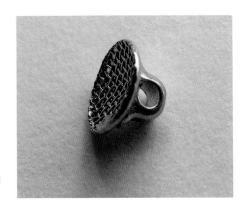

Figure 13.14 Eyelet. Source: Reproduced by kind permission of Alan Hall.

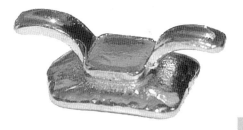

Figure 13.15 Cleat. Source: Reproduced by kind permission of Ortho-Care (UK) Ltd.

Archwires come in various sizes and fit into the channel in the bracket known as the slot. Initially, a very flexible fine archwire is placed that causes the teeth to move into alignment. Later on, heavier, more rigid archwires can then be used. Each orthodontist has their own preferred sequence of wire changes.

There are several materials from which wires are made:

- stainless steel (SS) (Figure 13.16)
- nickel titanium (NiTi)
- copper NiTi
- beta titanium.

They come in various cross-sections:

- round
- rectangular
- multi-stranded or braided, e.g. twist flex

and are supplied:

- pre-formed for upper and lower arches in a variety of shapes, either individually wrapped or in packets
- SS, NiTi and beta titanium, round and rectangular
- on spools (the length is cut off as required)
- in tubes, cut to length (monofilament, braided, coaxial, stranded wire).

The thickness (gauge) of wire ranges from very light to heavy and governs the amount of force being used.

FIXED APPLIANCES

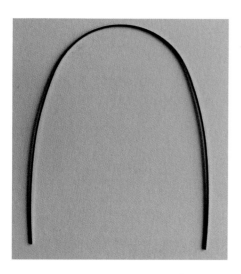

Figure 13.16 Stainless steel archwire. Source: Reproduced by kind permission of Alan Hall.

When they are fully engaged in the bracket slots and ligated or 'O-ringed' in, the force is then applied onto the tooth. When using self-ligating brackets, the same effect is achieved by closing the latch. When force is exerted by using auxiliaries such as springs or elastics, the archwire is usually passive.

When the teeth are well out of alignment, loops can be bent into the narrow-gauge SS archwire to give greater flexibility and speed up their movement. A light flexible wire can also be used in addition to the main wire as a 'piggy back' to engage a tooth that is too far outside the arch for the main wire to reach.

Coaxial wire

- has strands of wire wound around a core strand of wire.

Twist flex

- has three strands of wire wound together (e.g. popular as Wild Cat Wire).

Braided wire

- has eight strands of wire formed into a rectangular section wire.

Beta titanium wire

- can be formed into loops or bends
- is more flexible than SS
- is stronger than NiTi
- is nickel free.

FIXED APPLIANCES

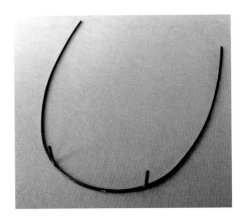

Figure 13.17 Posted archwire. Source: Reproduced by kind permission of Alan Hall.

Gold coated

- these are also available for patients with a nickel allergy in both round and rectangular sections.

Tooth coloured

- aesthetic wires in round and rectangular section (are coated with a tooth-coloured material).

Posted wires (Figure 13.17)

- these SS archwires have posts soldered to them to help when using traction, e.g. to close space.
- the posts can be shaped.
- the sizes are measured in millimetres between the posts along the anterior curve of the archwire.
- the upper wires range from 30 to 44 mm.
- the lower wire ranges from 24 to 28 mm.
- the wires are of rectangular section, usually 0.016 × 0.022 inches (0.41 × 0.56 mm), 0.018 × 0.025 inches (0.46 × 0.63 mm) or 0.019 × 0.025 inches (0.48 × 0.63 mm).

Reverse curve wire

Reverse curve wires (Figure 13.18), when placed on a flat surface, 'rock' so are not able to be stored in a conventional rack. These are inserted to:

- extrude teeth (mid arch)
- reduce an increase of overbite
- open the bite.

FIXED APPLIANCES

Australian wire

This round section wire (Figure 13.19):

- comes in either 10-inch (254 mm) lengths or spools of 25 feet (7.6 m)
- is cut as required
- is also popular when making bespoke archwires with bends and loops
- is supplied in several grades depending on what properties are needed, i.e. Regular, Regular Plus, Special and Special Plus, to fabricate the individual wire required.

Heat-activated wires

- many wires are now available as thermal wires
- they become activated at body heat.

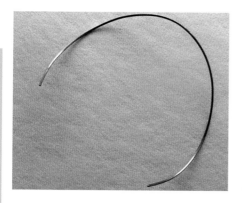

Figure 13.18 Reverse curve archwire. Source: Reproduced by kind permission of Alan Hall.

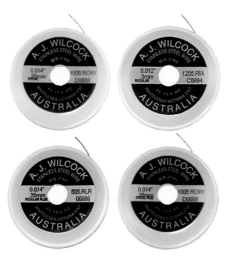

Figure 13.19 Australian wires. Source: Reproduced by kind permission of Ortho-Care (UK) Ltd.

FIXED APPLIANCES

Archwire storage

- archwires are kept in covered racks so that they are easily accessible (Figure 13.20).
- marking sticks are used to mark archwires. Because of cross-infection issues, these are single use.

Lingual archwires

- available in SS, NiTi, beta titanium and thermal wires
- shaped for lingual anatomy and to accommodate narrow inter-bracket dimensions.

Fixed retainer wire

These are wires specially made for cementing to the lingual surface of anterior teeth at debonding to assist with retention. This is often used when there is a high chance of relapse, e.g. where a wide midline diastema has been closed.

PLIERS

There are a great many pliers available for use with fixed appliance therapy. Just as every operator has their own favoured method of working, so they also have their preferred pliers and hand instruments. Frequently used ones include:

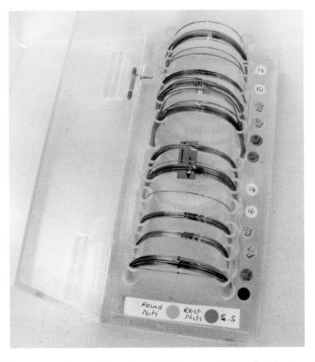

Figure 13.20 Archwire storage. Source: Reproduced by kind permission of Ortho-Care (UK) Ltd.

FIXED APPLIANCES

- safety-hold flush-cut distal end cutters (for trimming the end of archwire in the mouth)
- Weingart pliers
- pin and ligature cutters (for soft and narrow-gauge wire)
- light wire pliers
- Mathieu pliers
- mosquito forceps
- crown and band contouring pliers
- bird beak pliers
- Coon's pliers (for tying ligatures)
- step pliers (for making 'steps' in the wire, up or down)
- Tweed pliers (rectangular arch forming)
- Tweed loop-forming pliers
- torquing pliers
- hook crimping pliers
- NiTi cinch back pliers (to turn over the distal end of the archwire)
- bracket removing pliers
- posterior band removing pliers
- band slitter pliers
- adhesive removing pliers
- separating module pliers.

However, if you had too many of these on a tray, it would be:

- cluttered
- heavy
- require a lot of instruments
- considerable sterilising capability.

So, there are usually between four and six pliers per tray set-up, unless a specific procedure at a certain appointment calls for extra ones (Figure 13.21).

HAND INSTRUMENTS

In addition to pliers, several hand instruments are needed. Again, some are common to all procedures, others for specific uses only, such as fitting bands and brackets. Even if they are not normally needed, they must all be available and accessible in case of unforeseen treatment, e.g. breakages.

These include (Figure 13.22):

- ligature director
- plugger
- bite stick
- Mershon band pusher
- college tweezers
- mouth mirror

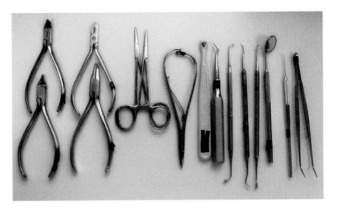

Figure 13.21 Sample fixed appliance tray set-up. Source: Reproduced by kind permission of Alan Hall.

- probe
- spatula
- Mitchell trimmer
- Wards carver
- flat plastic
- Twirl-On (for placing O-rings)
- Mathieu forceps
- mosquito forceps
- buccal tube tweezers
- direct bonding tweezers, straight or curved
- direct bonding tweezers with bracket aligner
- contra-angled handpieces and debonding burs
- direct bonding adhesive removing pliers.

AUXILIARIES

These are the items that are used in addition to bands, brackets and wires in the course of adjusting fixed orthodontic appliances (Figure 13.23). They include the following.

Ligatures

- these are available in several thicknesses.
- they can be pre-formed or open.
- a long ligature can be wound across many teeth over the wire as an alternative to O-rings:
  - can be placed to bridge a span to help support the archwire
  - can be used across many teeth under the wire to retain them, e.g. when they are not to be moved. This is known as a lace-up.
- individual short pre-formed ligatures (Quickligs) can also be used to hold an archwire securely in a bracket.

FIXED APPLIANCES

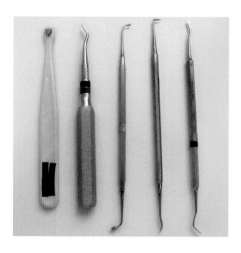

Figure 13.22 Bite stick, Mershon pusher, Mitchell trimmer and ligature director. Source: Reproduced by kind permission of Alan Hall.

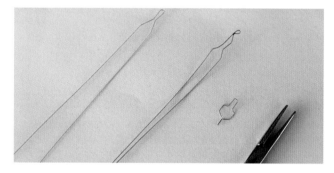

Figure 13.23 Ligature, Kobayashi ligature, Quicklig and mosquitos. Source: Reproduced by kind permission of Alan Hall.

- they are often used when greater strength is needed than an O-ring, e.g. severely rotated teeth.
- sometimes can be placed when a hook is needed, e.g. to attach elastics.

Elastic module chain

This is supplied on reels, either closed, short or openly spaced (Figure 13.24). Chain is:

- clear, grey or can be coloured (Figure 13.25)
- is used to apply force, e.g. for space closure, and lasts sufficiently between appointments.

Elastomeric modules (O-rings)

- these are used around the bracket to keep the archwire securely held.
- they are changed at each visit and at archwire adjustments.

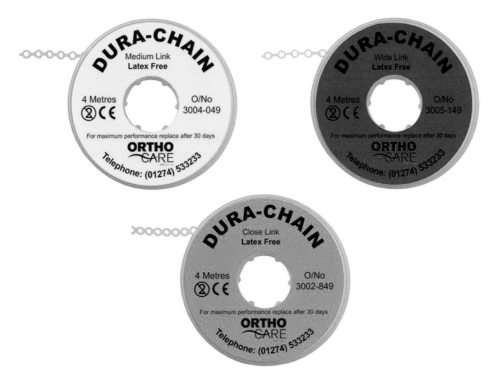

Figure 13.24 Narrow, medium and wide chain. Source: Reproduced by kind permission of Ortho-Care (UK) Ltd.

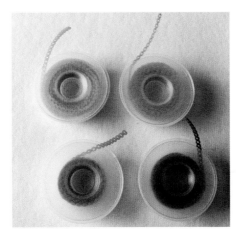

Figure 13.25 Coloured chain. Source: Reproduced by kind permission of Ortho-Care (UK) Ltd.

- they are put in place with Mathieu pliers or mosquito forceps (Figure 13.26).
- are often tied in 'figure of eight' for extra hold.
- they can be clear, white or black and in a wide range of colours (Figure 13.27).
- available in ivory to minimise staining from food, etc.

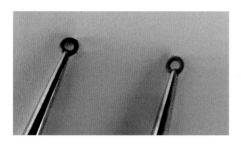

Figure 13.26 Elastomerics in mosquitos.

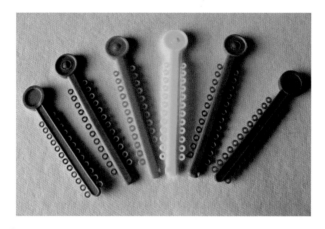

Figure 13.27 Range of coloured O-rings. Source: Reproduced by kind permission of Ortho-Care (UK) Ltd.

Protective sleeving

- this is placed over the archwire where there is a large space, e.g. an extraction site, to protect the inside of lip or cheek (Figure 13.28).
- used as a lip bumper (Figure 13.29) to protect soft tissues; easy to fit and remove.

Elastic string

- used to draw teeth together
- available in several strengths, e.g. Zing string.

Rotation wedges (Figure 13.30)

- small rubber wedges fitted under the archwire and attached under the tie wings of the bracket for rotating teeth
- e-link modules (Figure 13.31) connect brackets 'hook to hook' to rotate individual teeth
- available in a variety of sizes.

FIXED APPLIANCES

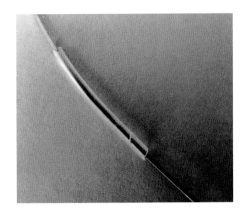

Figure 13.28 Archwire with sleeving. Source:
Reproduced by kind permission of Ortho-Care (UK) Ltd.

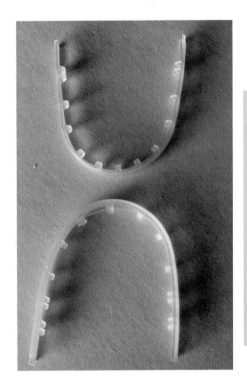

Figure 13.29 Protective bumper which fits over fixed
appliance brackets. Source: Reproduced by kind
permission of Ortho-Care (UK) Ltd.

FIXED APPLIANCES

NiTi power springs (Figure 13.32)

- can be used for opening and closing space
- are comfortable for patients
- provide a sustained force
- easier to keep clean, so aid oral hygiene
- reduce the frequency of visits.

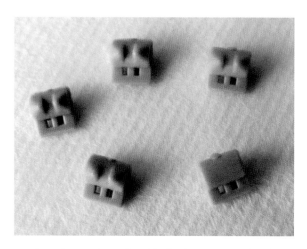

Figure 13.30 Rotation wedges. Source: Reproduced by kind permission of Ortho-Care (UK) Ltd.

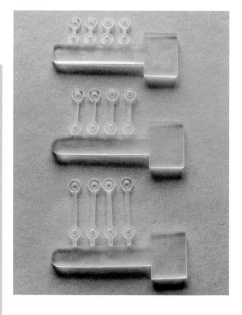

Figure 13.31 Space closing modules. Source: Reproduced by kind permission of Ortho-Care (UK) Ltd.

Coil (Figure 13.33)

This is supplied in spools and is cut to the length required. It comes in two forms, open and closed.

- open coil: used to open up spaces for accommodation of crowded teeth.
- closed coil: prevents a space from closing, e.g. post extraction.

Maxillary elastics (Figure 13.34)

- are fitted to attachments
- are worn vertically between the upper and lower arch
- are of varying strengths.

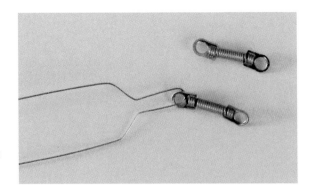

Figure 13.32 NiTi power springs. Source: Reproduced by kind permission of Ortho-Care (UK) Ltd.

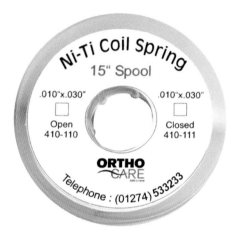

Figure 13.33 NiTi coil spring. Source: Reproduced by kind permission of Ortho-Care (UK) Ltd.

Elastic placer (Figure 13.35)

• with hooks at each end, this helps patients fit and remove their elastic bands.

Separating modules (Figure 13.36)

• come in two sizes, small for anterior placement, large for posterior
• smooth, often radiopaque
• are placed between teeth some days prior to fitting bands
• separating springs (Figure 13.37), not commonly used now, are useful for partially erupted teeth
• are made of metal
• are curved, designed to spring contact points apart
• are fitted between teeth using pliers.

A FIXED APPLIANCE TRAY

For the nurse it is helpful to have a standard 'tray set-up'. These trays can be assembled prior to a clinical session which saves time. The tray is made up of the instruments that the clinician likes and routinely uses.

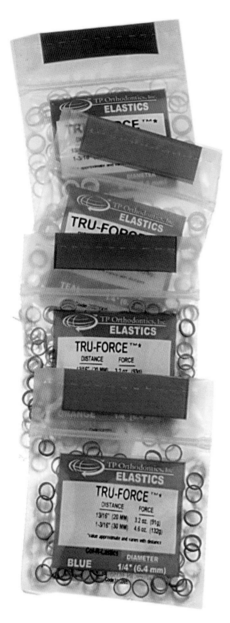

FIXED APPLIANCES

Figure 13.34 Intra-maxillary elastics.
Source: Reproduced by kind permission of TP
Orthodontics. True Force is registered trademark of TP
Orthodontics Inc. All rights reserved.

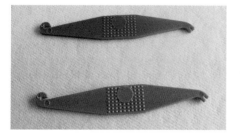

Figure 13.35 Elastic placer. Source: Reproduced by
kind permission of Ortho-Care (UK) Ltd.

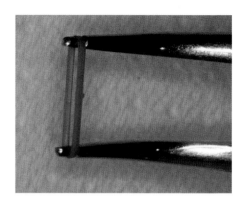

Figure 13.36 Separating module on plier. Source: Reproduced by kind permission of Jonathan Sandler.

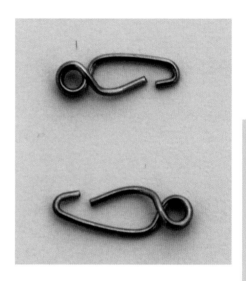

Figure 13.37 Separating springs. Source: Reproduced by kind permission of Ortho-Care (UK) Ltd.

A fixed appliance tray set-up might typically include the following popular choices.

Pliers (Figure 13.38)

- light wire cutters, for cutting soft wire and ligatures
- distal end cutters, for cutting off excess archwire behind the molars
- Weingart utility pliers to assist archwire insertion
- light wire pliers, for loops, cinching, etc.
- mosquito forceps
- Mathieu forceps for placing elastomerics, ligating and tying in.

Hand instruments

- mirror, probe and College tweezers
- Mitchell trimmers to locate brackets, remove adhesive, etc.
- Merton pusher/plugger to seat and contour molar bands

FIXED APPLIANCES

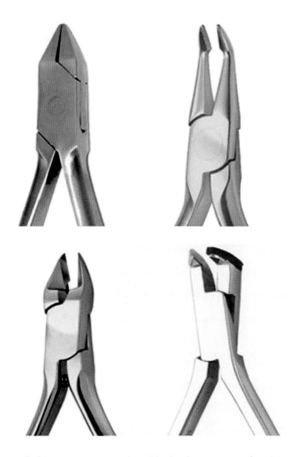

Figure 13.38 Selection of pliers. Source: Reproduced by kind permission of Ortho-Care (UK) Ltd.

- bite stick to seat bands
- director/ligature tucker to hold wire securely in bracket slot when ligating or turn under the 'pigtail' of excess wire
- dividers/rulers to measure widths between teeth or across the dental arch (Figure 13.39).

It is necessary, and many orthodontists consider it vital, that they have each patient's study models available for every appointment. When preparing to adjust a fixed appliance, it is always wise to have everything ready to:

- replace a lost bracket
- re-cement a loose band.

Therefore, you always need to have at hand:

- the light source
- adhesive
- cements.

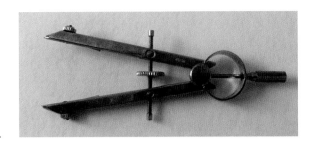

Figure 13.39 Dividers. Source: Reproduced by kind permission of Alan Hall.

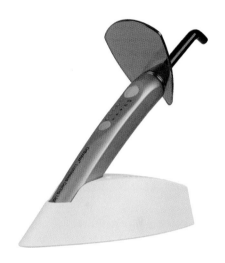

Figure 13.40 Ortholux™ luminous curing light. Source: Reproduced with permission of 3M Unitek © 2019. All rights reserved.

The orthodontic patient will sometimes present with a breakage which they do not know about. So:

- always have everything ready for every eventuality
- keep all the auxiliaries covered and within easy reach
- have the covered archwire stands nearby
- have the LED curing light always ready and charged (Figure 13.40)
- keep extra items in case they are needed, as it saves time changing gloves before searching in drawers or storage areas.

CEMENTS

There are several cements that are widely used in orthodontics (Figure 13.41):

- many leach fluoride
- some are a powder and liquid mixed and which set in time in the mouth
- some are powder and liquid which is light cured in the mouth.

FIXED APPLIANCES

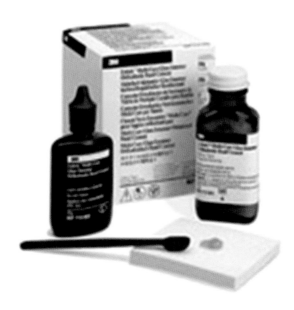

Figure 13.41 Cements. Source: Reproduced with permission of 3M Unitek © 2019. All rights reserved.

ADHESIVES

There are many orthodontic adhesives on the market, of which one is illustrated (Figures 13.42 and 13.43).

- some are ready mixed, dispensed straight from a syringe, and light cured.
- some come in two parts which need to be mixed together, e.g. base and catalyst.
- some are especially for use in bonding fixed retainers, and these tend to flow more easily.

If using light-cure adhesives when attaching clear brackets, the working time is reduced as the heat and light from the operating light will make it set more quickly, whereas metal brackets have to have the light applied to them from the side.

ETCHANT/PRIMER

Before fixing the bracket to the tooth, the enamel tooth surface must be prepared. This can be achieved by:

- using acid etch, washing and drying the tooth, and then applying primer
- using a system where this process is combined in a single application, known as self-etch primer (SEP) (Figure 13.44).

Single SEP doses are available as 'lollipops'. This system does not necessarily need a totally dry field.

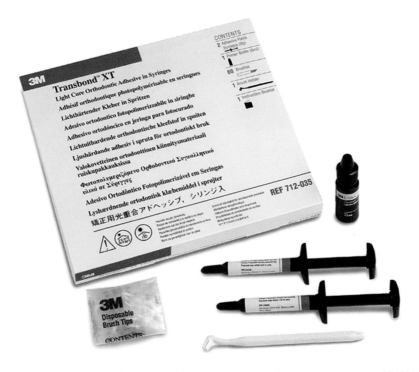

Figure 13.42 Transbond TX™ light curing adhesive. Source: Reproduced with permission of 3M Unitek © 2019. All rights reserved.

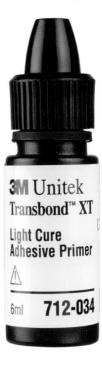

Figure 13.43 Transbond TX™ light curing primer. Source: Reproduced with permission of 3M Unitek © 2019. All rights reserved.

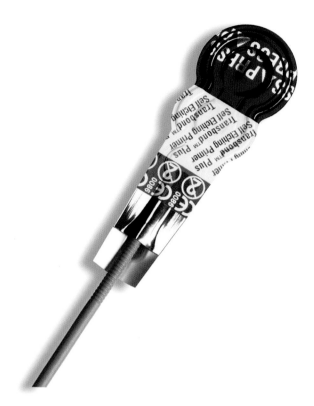

Figure 13.44 Transbond™ Plus self-etching primer. Source: Reproduced with the permission of 3M Unitek © 2019. All rights reserved.

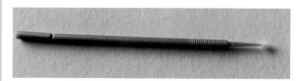

Figure 13.45 Microbrush. Source: Reproduced by kind permission of Ortho-Care (UK) Ltd.

MICROBRUSHES

Microbrushes (Figure 13.45):

- come in a variety of applicator sizes
- are useful when applying etchant or primer to teeth
- are single use.

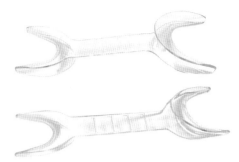

Figure 13.46 Mirahold™ lip retractors. Source: Reproduced by kind permission of TOC.

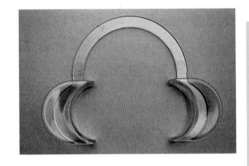

Figure 13.47 Lip retractors. Source: Reproduced by kind permission of TOC.

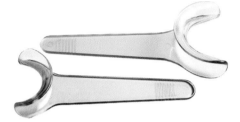

Figure 13.48 Cheek retractors. Source: Reproduced by kind permission of TOC.

LIP RETRACTORS

Lip retractors (Figures 13.46 and 13.47):

- are usually double-ended, and come in small, teenage and large sizes
- can be plastic or metal
- can be used when taking intra-oral photographs
- should be autoclavable.

CHEEK RETRACTORS

Cheek retractors (Figure 13.48):

- are all in one piece
- are made of plastic

FIXED APPLIANCES

- are used to keep the cheeks and lips away from the teeth when bonding
- should be autoclavable.

AIDS TO PATIENT COMFORT

Relief wax (Figure 13.49) comes in small boxes for patients to self-administer if the appliance is rubbing the inside of the lip/cheek.

Silicone (medical grade):

- stays in place more easily
- does not become brittle
- can be used to cover a larger area
- has no taste or smell
- unlike wax, it is not affected by heat.

Mouth gel:

- is a topical application for painful ulcers and abrasions
- quickly removes discomfort
- guards against infection
- must be non-salicylate containing (for children).

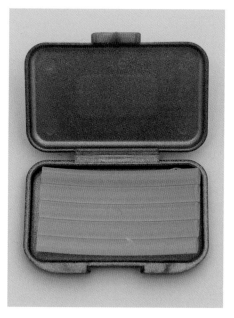

Figure 13.49 Relief wax. Source: Reproduced by kind permission of Ortho-Care (UK) Ltd.

INTERPROXIMAL REDUCTION

Interproximal reduction (IPR), which involves taking tiny amounts of enamel from mesial and distal contact points of teeth, may also be used in fixed appliance therapy:

- where it is necessary to de-rotate a single tooth
- if there is an area of very mild localised crowding
- to eliminate dark triangles
- to improve the shape of the papilla
- when re-shaping and re-contouring.

For more information on IPR, see Chapter 19.

As there are so many sharp wires and metal bands and brackets associated with these appointments, you must have a sharps bin nearby. You must know and be familiar with the appropriate policy to follow.

With what must seem an alarming array of equipment and consumables around you, it is time to start work. Every nurse has their own method of working and organising to keep one step ahead – anticipation is your third hand! It saves so much time and makes the day run more smoothly.

FIXED APPLIANCES

Chapter 14

Fixed appliances: direct bonding

There are two methods of fitting fixed appliances:

- direct bonding
- indirect bonding.

Direct bonding is used more routinely and this chapter aims to highlight the nurse's role in this process.
  Different clinicians work in different ways.

- some clinicians like to work 'four handed' with a nurse.
  - *This means that the nurse hands them the correct instrument at the appropriate time.*
  - *the nurse also cuts and hands them ligatures, chain, coil, etc.*
  - the tray is on the **nurse's side**, placed centrally on the bracket table/working area.
- some clinicians prefer to work from the tray themselves.
  - they select pliers, archwires, etc.
  - they cut their own chain, sleeving, etc.
  - *the nurse may load Mathieu pliers/mosquito forceps with elastomerics.*
  - the tray is on the **clinician's side**, placed centrally on the bracket table/working area.

NB It is important that at all appointments the patient's model box is available with the study models within reach. Models should be taken out of the box before the treatment begins and the nurse puts on gloves.

COMMUNICATION

Nurses also communicate with and monitor the patient:

- *ask them how they are*
- *ask them what's going on in their life, etc.*
- *ask them what colours of O-rings they want.*

Basic Guide to Orthodontic Dental Nursing, Second Edition. Fiona Grist.
© 2020 John Wiley & Sons Ltd. Published 2020 by John Wiley & Sons Ltd.

The orthodontist meanwhile refreshes their memory reading or writing up notes and so forth.

If the patient is sitting in silence, they are less likely to be brave enough to mention:

- *any concerns or problems they may have about their treatment or appliance*
- *any teasing that they may be experiencing*
- *that they have forgotten the rules, and have a breakage.*

ALLERGY AWARENESS

Orthodontic fixed appliance brackets are made of stainless steel which can contain nickel, chromium and cobalt. Archwires are also made of stainless steel and nickel titanium. It is important that any allergy to nickel should be recorded as part of the general medical history and clearly marked on the notes. This also applies to latex and rubber, which may be present in elastics and modules.

ORAL PIERCING

Many patients have oral piercings (Figure 14.1), and these can include:

- a discreet stud in the lip
- one or more large lip rings
- cheek studs
- unilateral or bilateral tongue studs.

The patient may or may not be asked to remove these during treatment. If required to remove their jewellery, the patient may need a mirror to take it out and replace it.

Patients need to be advised:

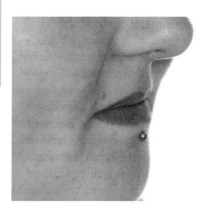

Figure 14.1 Lip stud. Source: Reproduced by kind permission of Jonathan Sandler.

FIXED APPLIANCES: DIRECT BONDING

- that there is a chance their metal jewellery might damage the appliance, e.g. if it is 'clicked' against a palatal arch
- that the metal might damage the teeth, especially the incisal edges
- that the metal could obstruct space closure sites
- that if sharp, the jewellery might puncture the clinician's glove.

LOCAL ANAESTHETIC

Local anaesthetic delivered by syringe is very rarely needed when fitting or adjusting appliances but topical anaesthetic may be used if required.

FITTING A FIXED APPLIANCE USING THE DIRECT BONDING TECHNIQUE

The patient has the molar bands and the brackets fitted onto each tooth individually. This can be done in four ways and depends on:

- the preferences of the clinician
- the age and capabilities of the patient
- fitting times in and around any dental extractions that are required.

Method 1

- the patient comes in to have the separators placed.
- at the next visit these are removed and the bands fitted and cemented.
- at the next visit the brackets are bonded.

Method 2

- the patient comes in to have the separators placed.
- a week later, they have the bands and brackets fitted in one visit.

Method 3

- the patient has the separators fitted at the same visit as the brackets.
- at the next appointment, they have the separators removed and the bands fitted and cemented.

Method 4

- the patient has upper and lower brackets but with buccal tubes bonded on all first molars instead of molar bands.

In cases where the patient is planned to have orthognathic surgery, bands are fitted to the first and usually second molars. In these patients, hooks can be incorporated into the brackets (Figure 14.2) on canine and premolar teeth. Some clinicians prefer to fit crimpable hooks directly onto the archwire prior to surgery.

When fitting brackets with composite adhesive material, a light source is used. It is important that the patient, orthodontist and nurse wear protective glasses (Figure 14.3) that have orange-tinted lenses at all times when they are curing bracket adhesive. No one must look directly at the blue light. Parents in the surgery must wear glasses too.

METHOD 1: THREE VISITS

First appointment: putting in the separators

The nurse needs to prepare:

- *the patient's clinical notes*
- *mouth mirror*
- *elastomeric separators*
- *separator placement pliers*
- *floss*
- *a follow-up appointment.*

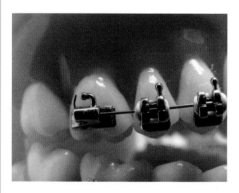

Figure 14.2 Hooks on brackets. Source: Reproduced by kind permission of Alan Hall.

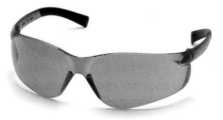

Figure 14.3 Safety glasses for use with LED light. Source: Reproduced by kind permission of TOC.

Procedure

The nurse needs to:

- *ensure that the patient and staff have appropriate personal protection*
- *make sure that the patient is seated comfortably*
- *establish which teeth are to be banded at the next visit as this indicates how many separators are needed*
- *give the clinician the separators of their choice, loaded on pliers*
- *after the separators are placed, explain to the patient:*

  - *that they may feel strange, like a piece of food has become wedged between their teeth*
  - *this feeling will go after a few hours, but some discomfort may be felt in these teeth for a day or two*
  - *they cannot use floss in molar areas while separators are in position*
  - *separators will do no harm should they be accidentally swallowed.*

Second appointment: fitting and cementing the bands

The nurse will need to prepare:

- *the patient's clinical notes*
- *model box*
- *mirror, probe and College tweezers*
- *prophylactic handpiece*
- *orthodontic prophylactic paste (oil-free)* (Figure 14.4)
- *rubber cup*
- *dental floss*
- *3-in-1 syringe*
- *suction*
- *cheek retractors*
- *cotton rolls*
- *cement, pad and spatula*
- *box of bands* (Figure 14.5) *and spare College tweezers*
- *posterior band remover*

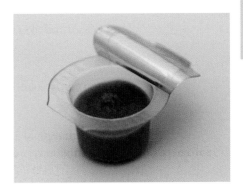

Figure 14.4 Orthodontic prophy paste. Source: Reproduced by kind permission of Ortho-Care (UK) Ltd.

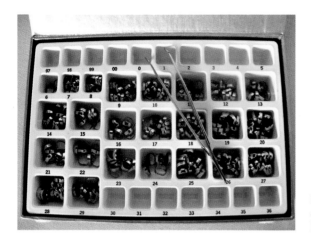

Figure 14.5 Box containing a selection of molar bands. Source: Reproduced by kind permission of Alan Hall.

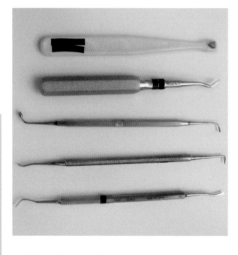

Figure 14.6 Bite stick, Mershon pusher, Mitchell trimmer and ligature director. Source: Reproduced by kind permission of Alan Hall.

- *Mershon pusher* (Figure 14.6)
- *plugger*
- *acrylic bite stick*
- *Mitchell trimmer*
- *patient relief wax or medical-grade silicone*
- *hand mirror.*

Procedure

- *the nurse ensures that:*
  - *there is a glass of mouthwash available (some cements taste bitter)*
  - *the patient and staff are using personal protective equipment*
  - *the patient is sitting comfortably in the chair (this is a longer appointment and younger patients can get restless and fidgety).*
- *the nurse gives the clinician a probe so that the separators can be removed.*
- the teeth are flossed.

- all the areas that are being treated are cleaned using a contra-angled handpiece, rubber cup and oil-free prophylactic paste.
- *the nurse gets the patient to rinse thoroughly or irrigates the mouth and aspirates.*
- using the study model as a guide for sizing, the clinician selects the appropriate molar bands for the teeth in question (these may be first molars, second molars or both)
- the bands are removed and dried.
- *the nurse ensures that there is a dry field in the mouth, using plenty of cotton rolls.*
- *the nurse mixes the cement and lines each band with it.*
- *these are handed individually to the clinician, with a Mershon pusher, plugger or bite stick, whichever is needed.*
- the clinician seats the bands on the teeth, asking the patient to bite on damp cotton wool rolls.
- excess cement is quickly wiped away with gauze or cotton wool roll, or left until nearly set and removed using a Mitchell trimmer or Wards carver.
- *the nurse then asks the patient to rinse again.*
- *the patient is given a hand mirror to see what the brace looks like and asked to check that there is nothing sharp or uncomfortable.*
- *the patient is given instructions on oral hygiene and dietary advice plus a box of wax or medical-grade silicone in case they have any problems with the appliance rubbing the cheeks and tongue.*
- *the patient is also given a leaflet and reminded what is to be done at the next appointment.*

Third appointment: fitting the brackets and archwires

The patient has the molar bands in place so the brackets are now fitted. (In adult patients where there are anterior crowns or veneers, it is sometimes necessary to use porcelain primer before bonding brackets to these teeth.)

The nurse needs to prepare:

- *the patient's clinical notes*
- *model box*
- *mirror probe and College tweezers* (Figure 14.7)
- *prophy handpiece*
- *rubber cups*
- *orthodontic oil-free prophy paste*
- *3-in-1 tips syringe*
- *saliva ejector*
- *LED curing light*
- *safety glasses for operators and patient*
- *orientation card of the brackets needed* (Figure 14.8)
- *if self-ligating brackets are used, the hand instrument for closing the bracket*
- *cheek retractors*
- *cotton wool rolls*
- *acid etch in disposable Dappen's pot* (Figure 14.9) *and microbrush*

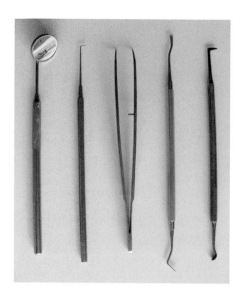

Figure 14.7 Mirror probe, College tweezers, ligature director and Mitchell trimmer. Source: Reproduced by kind permission of Alan Hall.

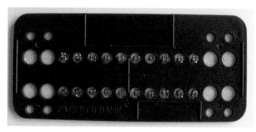

Figure 14.8 Orientation card. Source: Reproduced by kind permission of Alan Hall.

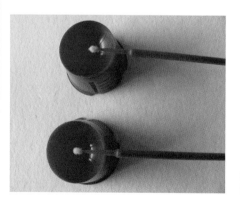

Figure 14.9 Acid etch and primer in Dappen's pots. Source: Reproduced by kind permission of Alan Hall.

FIXED APPLIANCES: DIRECT BONDING

- *primer in disposable Dappen's pot and microbrush, or self-etching primer (SEP) in 'lollipop' (Figure 14.10)*
- *light-curing adhesive (syringe or tube); not needed if using pre-coated brackets*
- *quickligs, for tying in individual teeth*
- *bracket-holding tweezers (Figure 14.11)*
- *Mitchell trimmer*
- *light wire pliers (Figure 14.12)*

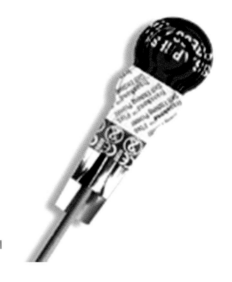

Figure 14.10 Transbond™ self-etching primer. Source: Reproduced by kind permission of 3M Unitek © 2019. All rights reserved.

Figure 14.11 Bracket-holding tweezers. Source: Reproduced by kind permission of Ortho-Care (UK) Ltd.

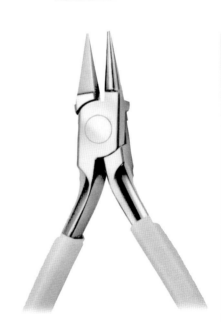

Figure 14.12 Light wire pliers. Source: Reproduced by kind permission of Ortho-Care (UK) Ltd.

- *Weingart pliers* (Figure 14.13)
- *light wire and pin ligature cutters* (Figure 14.14)
- *distal end cutters* (Figure 14.15)
- *Mathieu forceps* (Figure 14.16)
- *mosquito forceps* (Figure 14.17)
- *a selection of initial archwires*

FIXED APPLIANCES: DIRECT BONDING

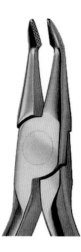

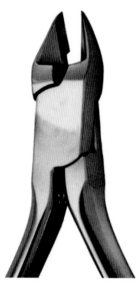

Figure 14.13 Weingart pliers. Source: Reproduced by kind permission of Ortho-Care (UK) Ltd.

Figure 14.14 Ligature and pin cutters. Source: Reproduced by kind permission of Ortho-Care (UK) Ltd.

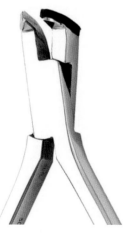

Figure 14.15 Distal end cutters. Source: Reproduced by kind permission of Ortho-Care (UK) Ltd.

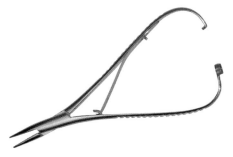

Figure 14.16 Mathieu forceps. Source: Reproduced by kind permission of Ortho-Care (UK) Ltd.

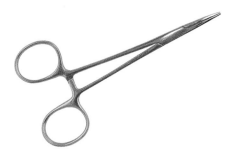

Figure 14.17 Mosquito forceps. Source: Reproduced by kind permission of Ortho-Care (UK) Ltd.

- *O-rings*
- *bumper sleeve (if needed to protect soft tissues adjacent to a wide span of wire)*
- *sharps box for excess trimmed wire*
- *hand mirror and brushes for oral hygiene instruction*
- *patient's instruction leaflet*
- *box of patient relief wax or medical-grade silicone.*

Procedure

- *the nurse ensures that clinician, patient and nurses have the appropriate personal protection.*
- *the patient is made comfortable.*
- *the patient selects their choice of coloured O-rings (Figure 14.18); this allows them to customise their appliance.*
- *check that there have not been any problems since the last visit.*
- *the brackets on their orientation tray are made ready.*
- *any brackets not needed (i.e. unerupted or extracted teeth) are removed from the tray.*
- *if the procedure uses the etch and prime method, etchant and primer in separate disposable Dappen's pot with microbrushes should be to hand.*
- *if an all-in-one system of SEP is being used, the 'lollipop' should be made ready.*
- all the surfaces to be treated are cleaned using a contra-angled prophylactic handpiece, rubber cup and some oil-free prophylactic paste.
- the teeth are washed thoroughly.
- *the patient should be allowed to rinse or should be aspirated.*
- a cheek retractor is fitted.
- the teeth are isolated and dried thoroughly.

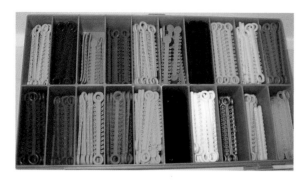

Figure 14.18 Box of coloured O-rings. Source: Reproduced by kind permission of Ortho-Care (UK) Ltd.

- a spot of etchant is placed on the labial surface of each tooth at bracket height.
- after brief period this is washed off.
- *aspirate and dry again.*
- *a spot of primer is placed onto the labial surface of each tooth at bracket height, using either of the following methods:*
  - *the base of the bracket is loaded with adhesive from the syringe, or*
  - *the pre-coated bracket is removed from its protective bubble wrapping.*

A number of bracket systems incorporate a method of holding the archwire in the bracket; these are known as self-ligating brackets (Figures 14.19 and 14.20). When using these you need a hand instrument to open and close the latch but do not need any elastomerics.

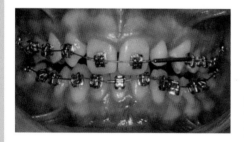

Figure 14.19 Self-ligating brackets (still with their identifying spots). Source: Reproduced by kind permission of Jonathan Sandler.

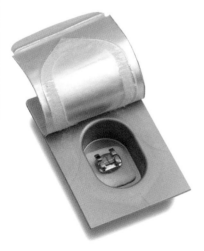

Figure 14.20 Advanced APC™ II bracket in open blister. Source: Reproduced with kind permission of 3M Unitek © 2019. All rights reserved.

FIXED APPLIANCES: DIRECT BONDING

- *the clinician should be handed the brackets on bracket-holding tweezers (when using SEP 'lollipops', once they have been activated and the tip of the microbrush becomes coated, it 'paints' the solution onto the surface of the tooth and the bracket is positioned).*

Keep doing this until all the brackets have been fitted in the quadrant/arch. It depends on clinical preference in which sequence you work and how many brackets are placed before light curing. Some clinicians cure every bracket individually, others will cure a quadrant, others an entire arch.

After all brackets are in position:

- *remove the cheek retractor and let the patient rest a minute (it will feel strange, so a word of encouragement will be helpful)*
- *then an archwire is selected and cut to just a little longer than the patient's arch length*
- the wire is first fitted into the molar tubes and then eased into the bracket slots
- the chosen O-rings are then placed.

The O-ring is placed over the archwire, around the outside rim of the bracket under the tie wings. Later wires might need to be tied in more tightly, so the O-ring is tied in a figure of eight or a metal ligature may be used.

Distal end cutting pliers are now used to cut off any excess wire distally that is protruding out of the buccal tube. If the wire is bendable, the clinician may choose instead to cinch the wire (i.e. turn the end towards the gingivae). This makes it harder for the archwire to slide out of the tube or to slew around to one side so that one end becomes too long and sticks into the patient's cheek.

- *check that the patient feels comfortable.*
- *give the patient oral hygiene instruction, demonstrating the special brushes, etc.*
- *explain the importance of following dietary advice.*
- *show them how to use the medical-grade silicone or relief wax and give them a box.*
- *demonstrate how to clean and look after the appliances.*
- *check they still have their original leaflet; if not, give them another one.*
- *show them themselves in the mirror.*

Your patient may need to have their confidence boosted a bit so:

- *admire their appliance and tell them they look great*
- *congratulate them, say what a good patient they have been*
- *remember that their mouth may feel weird and that they may feel anxious.*

Advise the patient that now the wires are starting to move all the teeth involved in the appliance, there will be some discomfort especially when chewing. To mitigate this, a soft diet and very small pieces of food are advisable. This may be necessary for a few days.

For some patients, the first experience of dental treatment is their orthodontics. For them it is a new experience and can be quite daunting.

Fixed appliance trays have all the equipment that may be needed; sometimes it is not all used but often it is (Figure 14.21).

FIXED APPLIANCES: DIRECT BONDING

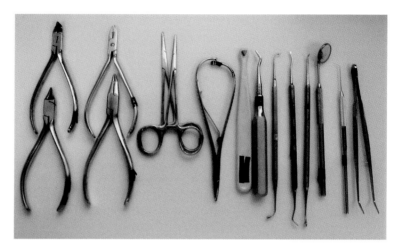

Figure 14.21 Sample fixed appliance tray. Source: Reproduced by kind permission of Alan Hall.

METHOD 2: TWO VISITS

This method has one very brief visit followed by a much longer one:

- separators
- brackets and bands fitted together.

This method uses the same layout for the initial separating appointments. At the next appointment, the bands and the brackets are fitted at the same time. This means all pliers and hand instruments from the bracket and band-fitting procedures must be available.

METHOD 3: TWO VISITS

This method involves two visits for:

- separators and brackets
- bands.

At the first appointment, separators are placed and then the brackets are fitted. At the second appointment, the separators are removed, the bands fitted and the archwires placed.

Patients sometimes accidentally lose a bracket; this can be repaired at the second visit.

METHOD 4: ONE VISIT

This method involves just one visit for:

- brackets and buccal tubes.

This is much the quickest method as there is no need for separation as no bands are fitted. When the brackets are fitted and buccal tubes fixed to all first molars, this is done in one continuous process. Some clinicians like to place and cure the buccal tubes first. They may do these individually if keeping the area dry is an issue.

Now that the patient's fixed appliance has been fitted and the active phase of treatment has begun, the teeth are on the move. Between now and de-bonding there will be many appointments.

Before the patient arrives at a routine adjustment appointment, you are never quite certain what problems the patient may have had. Sometimes they do not even know themselves if they have a broken archwire or a loose bracket. So, prepare for the expected and plan for the unexpected.

In addition to having the routine equipment necessary to adjust fixed appliances, it is helpful to have everything handy for the unexpected. As in most things, as you gain experience over a period of time you can plan ahead and anticipate what will be needed.

Also, many clinicians are creatures of habit. As the treatment progresses, they have a routine. They also work in the mouth in an established pattern, e.g. left to right or upper before lower arch. Getting to know these ways really helps. It keeps the nurse one step ahead and appointment times on track.

OTHER USES AND APPLICATIONS FOR FIXED APPLIANCES

Sectional fixed

It is also possible to have fixed appliances that are:

- small
- localised
- sectional.

These are used if there is a specific isolated problem. It may involve only a few brackets, e.g. uprighting a tipped molar prior to bridgework.

Additional 'piggyback' archwires

Sometimes, when the archwire is placed, there is a tooth which is just too far out of alignment for the archwire to lie in the bracket slot to be engaged. When this happens a small auxiliary wire is used which is placed alongside the main wire. This is known as a piggyback wire. It is ligated in alongside the main wire but has the flexibility to engage the outreach tooth into a position which will enable it to be eventually included into the main wire.

FIXED APPLIANCES: DIRECT BONDING

Chapter 15

Fixed appliances: indirect bonding and lingual orthodontics

This chapter is an extension of the two previous ones that dealt with fixed appliances which were directly bonded onto the labial surface of the teeth.

However, attachments can also be bonded onto the teeth using an indirect method. This is a technique that is frequently used when bonding attachments to lingual surfaces.

LINGUAL ORTHODONTICS

The lingual technique (Figure 15.1) is becoming more widely used as patients are increasingly aware of the advantages and possibilities that it offers. Many clinicians are now practised in the technique and are able to offer it to their patients. It is an alternative to conventional fixed appliances that are fixed to the labial aspect of the teeth.

Lingual orthodontics was initially pioneered in the 1970s in Japan, where it was intended as an alternative for patients who took part in martial arts, and in America, where it was seen as an aesthetic option.

However, development was slow. The 1980s saw the introduction of aesthetic brackets and invisible aligners, which offered patients another, less visible, alternative to metal brackets.

Advantages

- of particular benefit to patients who play musical instruments by mouth, especially clarinets and saxophones.
- offer good aesthetics, especially for adults in occupations where appearance is an important consideration.

Disadvantages

- patients sometimes have difficulties with speech.
- there can be trauma to edges of the tongue (ulceration).
- it can be technically more challenging for the orthodontist.

Basic Guide to Orthodontic Dental Nursing, Second Edition. Fiona Grist.
© 2020 John Wiley & Sons Ltd. Published 2020 by John Wiley & Sons Ltd.

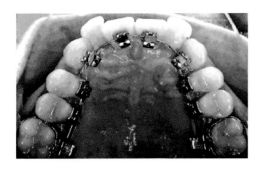

Figure 15.1 Lingual appliance. Source: Reproduced by kind permission of Paul Ward, British Lingual Orthodontics Society.

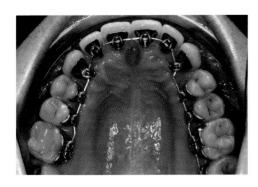

Figure 15.2 Lingual appliance with gold brackets. Source: Reproduced by kind permission of Paul Ward, British Lingual Orthodontic Society.

What materials are used

Because of their position in the mouth, the pliers and hand instruments that would be used to fit and adjust labial appliances would be of little use with lingual appliances. They need to have very fine edges that allow easy access to the brackets and give a less restricted view into the mouth. Impression materials are usually rubber based and models are cast in stone or a hard material.

Brackets

For ease of use, many lingual appliances use self-ligating brackets (Figure 15.2), but there are systems available which require ligatures or elastomerics. Black elastomerics are more visible and easier to locate in the lingual area of the mouth.

For the same reason, many of these appliances are fitted using the indirect bonding technique but some, notably those which concentrate on the anterior segment only, use direct bonding.

To accommodate the lingual surface, brackets tend to be smaller and the bases more curved.

Wires

The main difference between labial and lingual archwires is shape. Lingual archwires look rather like mushrooms as they have a rounded top which fits around the anterior teeth and then a 'bend' inwards to accommodate the differing canine/premolar width before flaring to attach to the premolars and molars (Figure 15.3).

Wires come as upper and lower, in the following sizes:

Round
0.010 inch (0.25 mm)
0.012 inch (0.30 mm)
0.013 inch (0.33 mm)
0.014 inch (0.36 mm)
0.016 inch (0.41 mm)

Square
0.016 × 0.016 inch (0.41 × 0.41 mm)
0.017 × 0.017 inch (0.43 × 0.43 mm)

Rectangular
0.016 × 0.022 inch (0.41 × 0.56 mm)
0.017 × 0.025 inch (0.43 × 0.63 mm)

Wires are available as:

- small
- medium
- large.

Wires are placed using a lingual wire placer (Figure 15.4).

Pliers

- ligature cutters are available with 40, 50 or 60° of angulation and have reversed or regular curves depending on where they are to be used.
- Mathieu pliers are curved.
- Weingart pliers have a 60° angle.
- bracket-removing pliers and cinch back pliers are of a special design.
- distal end cutters must be safety hold (Figures 15.5 and 15.6).

When a patient requires extractions as part of their treatment plan, it is usual to have this done a week prior to the fitting of the appliances. When the patient is having a lingual appliance fitted using the indirect technique, the appliance is fitted before the extractions

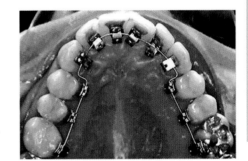

Figure 15.3 Lingual appliance: note shape of archwire. Source: Reproduced by kind permission of Paul Ward, British Lingual Orthodontic Society.

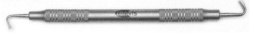

Figure 15.4 Lingual wire placer. Source: Reproduced by kind permission of TOC.

FIXED APPLIANCES

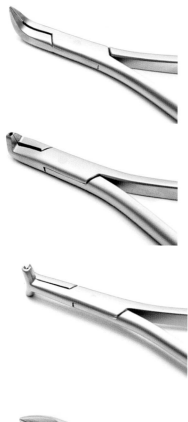

Figure 15.5 Lingual angled distal end cutter, lingual distal end cutters, lingual NiTi distal cinch back pliers. Source: Reproduced by kind permission of TOC.

FIXED APPLIANCES

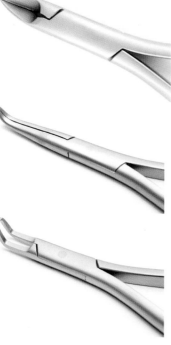

Figure 15.6 Lingual Weingart pliers, lingual debonding pliers and lingual light wire cutters. Source: Reproduced by kind permission of TOC.

are carried out. The archwire is removed to allow the dentist access for the extractions. This is to prevent the teeth adjacent to the extraction sites from moving between the time of extraction and fitting of the appliance.

Oral hygiene

Oral hygiene techniques when wearing lingual appliances have many similarities to those used when wearing labial appliances. To help maintain a healthy mouth, the following are all used:

- a toothbrush
- an interspace (tufted spiral) brush
- floss
- disclosing tablets
- mouthwash.

Toothbrush
For the anterior teeth, use the same technique as you would with labial bonding. Using a circular motion, make the tips of the bristles remove the plaque from the gingival margins towards the occlusal or incisal areas.

Interspace brush
The interspace brush is intended for use after brushing with the conventional toothbrush. It is intended to clean interdentally and, if the main brush is too big, to get into the crevices between the brackets.

Floss
Because it is more difficult to reach the brackets, it is helpful to use the long ready-cut lengths of floss that are stiffened at each end and have an area of thick 'furry' floss in the middle. The stiffened end is threaded under the archwire, and using a 'sawing' action it goes interproximally and under the gingiva and clears any residual plaque.

Disclosing tablets or solution
It is difficult to see the areas that may be being missed when brushing, so advise the patient to use a disclosing tablet or solution which contains coloured dye. By chewing the tablet, or rinsing with the liquid, the dye mixes with the saliva in the mouth and stains any areas of plaque. This makes it easier to see and be removed by further brushing. Patients may need a mouth mirror to see the lingual surfaces when they look in the bathroom mirror.

Mouthwash
As with labial fixed appliances, it is recommended that the patient uses a fluoride mouthwash every day.

Wax
Sometimes the brackets or attachments may feel uncomfortable and irritate the tongue. If this happens, strips of either silicone or wax can be used. This gives temporary relief and

FIXED APPLIANCES

allows the soft tissues to heal, as the irritation is masked. It is best to apply this, after brushing the teeth, as follows:

- using a piece of gauze or some cotton wool, dry the surface of the bracket
- take a section of wax or silicone and press it gently over the bracket (this acts as a buffer, making the mouth feel temporarily more comfortable).

Fitting a lingual appliance

Lingual appliances are nearly always bonded using the indirect method, with either a chemical cure or light-cured adhesive.

THE INDIRECT BONDING TECHNIQUE

Indirect bonding has been in use for many years, but in that time direct bonding onto the labial surface of the tooth has been more commonly used. However, indirect bonding of fixed appliances is now becoming more widely used. The patient still has attachments bonded onto their teeth but this uses a different method.

Indirect bonding suffered some issues in the initial stages, which have now largely been resolved with advances in specialty adhesives, refinement of transparent thermoplastic trays and customised guidelines for bracket placements. These have overcome some of the disadvantages, which included:

- difficulty in accessing malaligned teeth
- locating precise bracket position might be difficult as hard to see
- attachment becoming dislodged and so be incorrectly sited during bonding.

The main difference between the two techniques is that:

- direct bonding involves the clinician precisely placing each bracket on the tooth
- indirect bonding involves all the brackets being incorporated into a transfer tray after accurate placement is made on a model.

Indirect bonding usually involves fabrication of the tray by a dental technician. The clinician will send the work to be done to:

- an outside specialist laboratory
- an in-house technician
- a member of the dental team who has been trained in the technique.

It is important that the clinician fills in a detailed laboratory request form, which must include:

- whether it is for labial or lingual appliances
- for upper or lower, or both
- a full arch or a sectional one
- the type of brackets to be used

- information on any teeth not to be bonded
- any over-corrections that may be needed
- whether there is to be any interproximal stripping, and if so where and how much
- which type of bonding trays are needed
  - vacuum moulded (clear thermoplastic)
  - hard acrylic or silicone (if a two-tray system is used).

Some technicians use computer programs to calculate the bracket positions on teeth. Others use the work model, and a grid using vertical height and long axis lines drawn by pencil on the tooth.

There are several techniques employed in indirect bonding. Some methods use a single bonding tray and others use a flexible inner bonding tray with a rigid covering tray over that.

The one-tray bonding method using chemical cure adhesive

Prior to the fitting appointment

- the clinician would have taken rubber-based impressions of the teeth.
- these would go to the laboratory to be cast.
- a detailed instruction sheet would be given to the technician.
- on the working model, measurements were made to accurately position the bracket on each tooth.
- brackets were attached to the teeth on the model.
- a thermoplastic tray was made over these.
- the tray was removed with the brackets remaining *in situ*.

Fitting appointment

For the fitting appointment, the nurse needs to prepare:

- *clinical notes*
- *the bonding trays and work models*
- *mouth mirror*
- *probe and two pairs of College tweezers*
- *acetone in container*
- *adhesive (in two pots)*
- *frozen holder to keep them as cold as possible*
- *Dappen's pot*
- *microbrushes*
- *sandblasting equipment*
- *etchant*
- *dry field system*
- *3-in-1 tips*
- *cotton wool rolls*
- *pledgets*
- *contra-angled handpiece and rose-head burs*

- *scalers*
- *floss*
- *mouthwash and tissues*
- *hand mirror*
- *relief wax or medical-grade relief silicone*
- *instruction leaflets.*

Procedure at the fitting appointment

- *the nurse ensures that the dentist, patient and nurse have personal protective equipment.*
- the clinician tries in and checks the trays.
- *the nurse will then clean the trays with acetone.*
- the clinician then sandblasts the 'fitting' surfaces of individual teeth (each tooth takes 3–4 seconds).
- *the patient then thoroughly rinses and the nurse aspirates to clear the mouth.*
- the clinician attaches a dry field system (if both arches are being treated, the lower arch is done first).
- acid etch is applied by the clinician and removed after 30 seconds by the clinician, who then inserts cotton wool rolls and dries the mouth and all tooth surfaces.
- *at this point the nurse removes adhesive from the fridge (once removed from the fridge, the chemical cure adhesive must be kept cool, so the two containers are placed into the very cold container for the pots).*
- *the nurse puts four drops of each fluid in two Dappen's pots, mixing together with a microbrush.*
- *the nurse coats the base of the brackets with this solution.*
- the clinician paints the surfaces of the teeth.
- the tray is inserted firmly and held until the excess solution has set hard, usually in around 3 minutes.
- leaving this in place, the procedure may be repeated on the upper teeth.
- the trays are then taken out and all residual excess material removed with scalers.
- using articulating paper, the occlusion is checked for premature contact points.
- archwires, with ligatures or elastomerics, are placed.
- *the nurse gives the patient dietary advice and oral hygiene instructions.*
- *either silicone or relief wax is given to the patient in case of discomfort.*

The two-tray bonding method using light-cured adhesive

Prior to the fitting appointment

- a laboratory request would have been filled in and sent to the technician along with rubber-based impressions of the arch/arches to be bonded.
- the models were cast.
- the technician calculated and marked the site of the bracket placement.

- a bracket was attached onto each required tooth on the model with adhesive (this adhesive will form a custom-made base for the bracket so when it is bonded to the tooth, only a small amount of adhesive will be necessary).
- a thermoplastic flexible bonding tray was pressure formed.
- a rigid acrylic tray was then made which fitted over the flexible one.

Fitting appointment

For the fitting appointment, the nurse needs to prepare:

- *the patient's clinical notes*
- *bonding trays and working models*
- *tray set-up*
- *sandblasting equipment*
- *contra-angled handpiece and pumice/prophylactic paste*
- *rubber cup/wheel*
- *dry field system for moisture control which incorporates a cheek retractor*
- *LED light*
- *yellow protective glasses and hand-held shield*
- *either self-etching primer (SEP) as a 'lollipop' or etchant and primer in Dappen's pots with separate microbrushes*
- *3-in-1 aspirator tips*
- *adhesive*
- *cotton wool rolls*
- *cotton pledgets*
- *contra-angled handpiece and rose-head bur*
- *Miller's articulating forceps*
- *articulating paper*
- *hand mirror*
- *relief wax or medical-grade silicone*
- *information and instruction leaflets.*

Procedure at the fitting appointment

- *the nurse needs to ensure that the dentist, nurse and patient wear personal protective equipment.*
- *the patient should be seated comfortably.*
- the clinician inserts a moisture control and cheek retraction system (as with all bonding procedures, good moisture control is vital).
- arches are usually prepared and fitted one at a time, lowers first.
- teeth are cleaned with pumice or prophylactic paste using a contra-angled handpiece and a rubber cup (some clinicians also use etchant).
- after thorough spraying, the area is dried.
- the bases of the brackets are coated with adhesive enhancer.
- adhesive is then placed over that.
- the etched teeth are coated with sealant.
- adhesive is placed into the bracket base.

- with both flexible and rigid trays together, they are inserted onto the teeth from the back to the front of the mouth.
- use an LED light to set adhesive (ensure that protective yellow glasses are worn by all, including any parent or accompanying person in the room).
- the rigid tray is removed.
- using a scaler the flexible tray is cut and peeled away.
- after checking that the bracket channels are clear, the archwires are inserted.

If the appliance is placed lingually, the clinician must check that there is no occlusal interference. If there is, check with articulating paper held in Miller's forceps, and grind high spots using contra-angled slow handpiece and rose-head bur.

As the use of the indirect bonding technique for both lingual and labial appliances becomes more popular, an increasing number of dental team members are extending their skills and training within their units or practices, and now mark the models, position the brackets and construct the bonding tray. Nurses, trained by their clinician, can do the preparation in-house that would previously have been sent to the laboratory. This skill opens the way for an extended role for the nurse both in the preparation and fitting of the appliance.

Chapter 16

Ectopic canines

WHAT IS AN ECTOPIC CANINE?

The answer is that it is a perfectly normal canine tooth, but the clue is in the word 'ectopic'. The dictionary definition of this word is 'an abnormal location or position occurring congenitally or as a result of an obstruction or injury'. So, a canine tooth erupting in the wrong place is not good news for either the patient or the orthodontist!

Normally, teeth erupt in sequence.

- the permanent molars erupt distal to the deciduous dentition.
- incisors, canines and premolar teeth erupt into the space left by the exfoliated deciduous teeth.

An approximate guide to molar eruption is:

- first molars (the 6s) at 6 years
- second molars (the 7s) at 12 years
- third molars (the 8s) between 18 and 25 years.

THE PROBLEM

Eruption is usually straightforward but occasionally a tooth fails to erupt because:

- the root of the deciduous tooth does not resorb and stays firm
- the permanent tooth is deflected and is late in eruption or remains unerupted
- the required space is lost and it stays unerupted, impacted or erupts out of alignment
- the presence of a supernumerary tooth impedes the eruption of a permanent tooth, e.g. a central or lateral incisor.

If a tooth remains unerupted and out of position, it is said to be ectopic, a specific diagnostic term for a tooth following an incorrect path of eruption. This causes problems, and the teeth which are most likely to fail to erupt because they are off course, other than third

Basic Guide to Orthodontic Dental Nursing, Second Edition. Fiona Grist.
© 2020 John Wiley & Sons Ltd. Published 2020 by John Wiley & Sons Ltd.

(a)   (b)

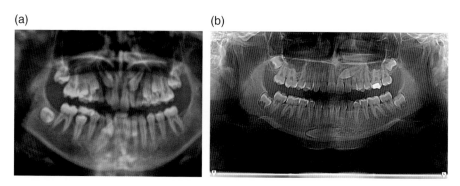

Figure 16.1 (a, b) Radiographs of ectopic canines. Sources: (a) Reproduced by kind permission of Alan Hall. (b) Reproduced by kind permission of Jo Clark.

molars, are the upper canines. This is more common in females than males and is a condition that can be inherited.

The upper canine begins its development high in the maxilla and has a longer distance than any other tooth in the dentition to travel before it erupts. More than three-quarters of ectopic canines lie palatally to the dental arch.

By about 10 years of age there is usually a bulge which can be palpated in the buccal sulcus to indicate that the tooth is on line. If it is not, then the dentist needs to monitor the progress of the tooth. Radiographs are taken in order to see just where it is and why it may not be erupting (Figure 16.1). Radiographs also show whether the crown of the permanent tooth is impacting into the roots of nearby incisors.

Although this may be damaging, it is a painless process. Sometimes the first sign that the ectopic tooth is in contact with, and has severely damaged the root of, a neighbouring tooth is that the tooth with the damaged root becomes mobile. This can happen quite rapidly and may possibly result in the loss of this tooth. Because they are adjacent to the canines, the damaged tooth is often the lateral incisor.

The orthodontist needs to know exactly where the unerupted tooth is lying in relation to the adjacent teeth, so the dentition needs to be assessed in all three planes. Thus the unerupted tooth may be:

- palatal (in the palate)
- labial (on the cheek side of the alveolus)
- occasionally across the dental arch bucco-lingually
- horizontal and high and near the apices of the adjacent teeth.

Clinical examination determines the location of the unerupted tooth. The area must be palpated buccally and palatally. The angle of the adjacent lateral may give a clue to the position of the canine and if it is mobile it could be due to root resorption. A buccal canine is often palpable but this is rare in the case of a palatal canine.

Radiographic examination uses the parallax technique. The word 'parallax' is defined as follows:

when an object appears to change its position because the person or instrument observing it has changed their position

or

how the position or direction of an object appears to differ when viewed from different positions, e.g. through the viewfinder and the lens of a camera

Horizontal Method:

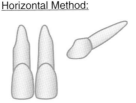
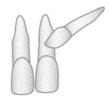

| 1. OPT and/or upper anterior occlusal; Impacted UL3 | 2. Lateral oblique occlusal, or peri-apical; Moved **horizontally** in the direction of the tube, so palatal to standing teeth | 3. Lateral oblique occlusal, or peri-apical; Moved **opposite** to the tube so is buccal |

Vertical Method:

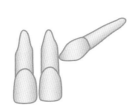
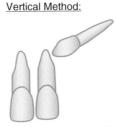
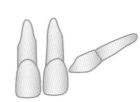

| 4. OPT; Impacted UL3 | 5. Upper anterior occlusal, UL3 moved **upward** with vertical shift of tube so is palatal | 6. Upper anterior occlusal, UL3 has moved **opposite** to the tube and so is buccal |

Figure 16.2 Diagram explaining parallax. Source: Reproduced by kind permission of Alan Hall.

This technique needs an orthopantomogram (OPT) and an upper occlusal or two peri-apical films taken from different angles. When these films are viewed side by side, i.e. OPT and upper occlusal (vertical) and OPT and upper occlusal (horizontal):

- the upper canine will appear to have moved with the X-ray tube if it is palatal
- the upper canine will appear to move in the opposite direction if it is buccal.

Figure 16.2 explains parallax and should make the phenomenon easier to understand.

Another method involves cone beam CT which, as it becomes more widely available, will become the diagnostic imagery of choice. It has the advantage of being able to the view the impacted tooth in three rather than two dimensions (Figures 16.3 and 16.4).

If the canine is not severely displaced, then the extraction of the retained deciduous canine may often provide sufficient space to encourage its permanent successor to erupt. However, these canine teeth sometimes:

- remain unerupted and buried in the maxilla
- occasionally erupt into the palate.

Ectopic and/or unerupted canines are much rarer in the mandible than the maxilla.

Treatment to retrieve these teeth can take many months and the patient has to be cooperative and understand that the treatment will take longer, especially if other features of a malocclusion have to be treated as well.

ECTOPIC CANINES

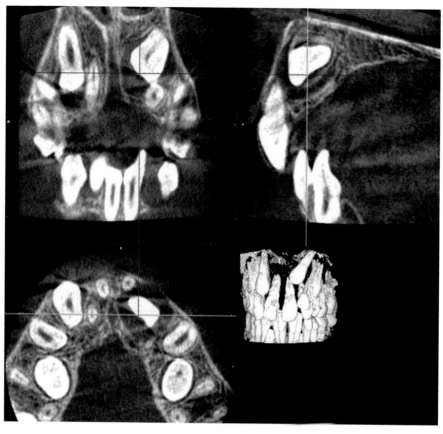

Figure 16.3 Cone beam CT images. Source: Reproduced by kind permission of Daljit Gill.

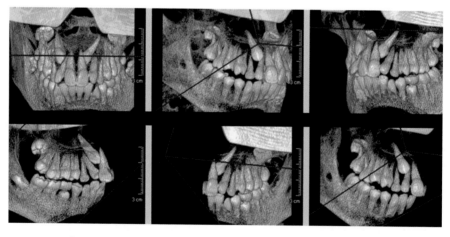

Figure 16.4 Cone beam CT images. Source: Reproduced by kind permission of Jonathan Sandler.

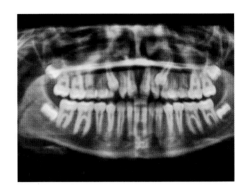

Figure 16.5 Radiograph of bilateral upper ectopic canines in an older child. Source: Reproduced by kind permission of Alan Hall.

If a patient has not been referred at the correct age (about 11 years old) and has a retained upper C by the time they are in their mid-teens (Figure 16.5), they have a dilemma that may have to be resolved by:

- leaving the deciduous tooth *in situ* and waiting for it to finally fail
- having it extracted and replaced with a bridge or implant
- having it extracted and seeking an orthodontic solution to retrieve the permanent tooth.

To bring the tooth into position requires the uncovering of the ectopic canine, which necessitates a surgical procedure, usually under general anaesthetic (GA), and the attachment of a bracket and gold chain as part of a fixed appliance. An orthodontic solution may mean that the patient could still be wearing fixed appliances long after their peers have had their fixed appliances removed.

If the patient decides to proceed with an orthodontic solution, a treatment plan is made also taking into account other features of the malocclusion.

CLINICAL INTERVENTION: WHAT THE TREATMENT INVOLVES

- a small surgical procedure exposes the buried tooth (usually under GA) (Figure 16.6).
- a 'window' is cut in the palatal or buccal soft tissues, or a flap is raised, and any bone over the buried tooth is removed.
- a gold-plated eyelet, often with chain or a bracket, is attached to the tooth.
- the wound is packed and the site is sutured, with the chain, if fitted, visible.
- if a flap was raised, this is closed over the surgical site, with the gold chain perforating the mucosa in the planned canine site.
- the free end of the gold chain can be temporarily cemented to an adjacent tooth with composite or sutured to the mucosa.

This attachment provides a 'handle' that can be used to attach wire, linked chain, elastic string, etc. to apply traction to begin to gently pull on the tooth. Light force must be used. This traction is usually applied in conjunction with a fixed appliance on the standing teeth; after each visit, as the tooth comes near to alignment, the number of links of gold chain can be reduced. Shorter and more frequent appointments are needed to renew the traction.

ECTOPIC CANINES

Sometimes the canine is rotated 180°, so that the buccal aspect is facing the palate for example. The tooth may need to be de-rotated, which can be a slow procedure that involves repositioning the bracket as the tooth de-rotates. This extends treatment time and can adversely affect the patient's compliance.

If the patient is not prepared to persist with wearing their appliance to allow time for this to be done, it is sometime possible to reach a compromise. By shaping the tooth and adding composite to the palatal surface, the tooth can be disguised to look as if it is the correct way round. This can give a good aesthetic result and is often more acceptable to the patient than additional months of traction to rotate the canine.

If the exposed tooth is lying buccally, there are two methods of treatment.

- a fixed appliance can be used, maybe needing a piggyback wire initially before being incorporated into the main archwire when it comes into a better alignment.
- less frequently, a removable appliance (Figure 16.7) can be used as a preliminary to a fixed appliance.

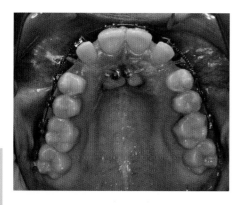

Figure 16.6 Surgically exposed palatal canines. Source: Reproduced by kind permission of Jonathan Sandler.

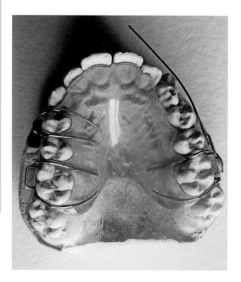

Figure 16.7 Upper removable appliance with untrimmed whip arm. Source: Reproduced by kind permission of Alan Hall.

ECTOPIC CANINES

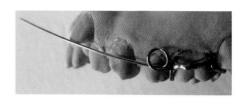

Figure 16.8 Untrimmed whip arm. Source: Reproduced by kind permission of Alan Hall.

A metal whip arm (Figure 16.8) from the crib of the removable appliance is positioned at the top (gingival side) of the bracket. This can be either a bracket into which the wire arm can slot or a 'blob' of composite which has had a groove indented into it. This could have the wire fitted into it and, if necessary, an elastomeric could secure it in place. The whip puts a force on the bracket and extrudes the tooth.

However, in nearly all cases fixed appliances are now used to retrieve ectopic canines.

Preparation

The nurse needs to prepare a fixed tray set-up:

- *the patient's model box*
- *mirror, probe and College tweezers*
- *light wire cutters*
- *light wire pliers*
- *distal end cutter*
- *Weingart plier*
- *ligature tuckers*
- *Mathieu pliers/mosquito forceps*
- *Coon's ligature locker pliers*
- *ruler*
- *dividers*
- *cheek retractor*
- *topical local anaesthetic, if needed*
- *3-in-1 tip*
- *fine aspirator tip.*

Depending on the preference of the clinician:

- *ligature wire*
- *spool elastic*
- *elastic links (chain)*
- *coil springs*
- *ligatures*
- *elastomerics (O-rings)*
- *cotton wool rolls*
- *Mitchell's trimmer*
- *sharps box*
- *archwire stands*
- *patient relief wax*

ECTOPIC CANINES

- *medical-grade relief silicone*
- *hand mirror.*

In some cases, a bracket that is bonded to the exposed canine does not have gold chain attached. *When this happens, it is vital to make sure that the appointment to attach the ligature, elastic or chain is organised as soon after the surgical pack is removed as possible.* If the soft tissues heal over the exposed tooth, this may prevent access and, in the worst cases, the patient may have to undergo another surgical procedure.

Where there is difficulty with access or vision, the clinician will sometimes make an eyelet from 0.012-inch ligature wire and pass the wire through the bracket channel as an easier way of fixing traction to the bracket.

Procedure

- *the nurse needs to assist the clinician at the chairside:*
  - *to ensure the patient and staff are wearing personal protection*
  - *the patient is made comfortable.*
- a cheek retractor is inserted
- using a 3-in-1 tip and aspirating, the wound is checked by the clinician to make sure that the pack has been fully removed and the bracket is clear of any obstruction.
- *the wound area is prone to bleeding, especially on the first visit when the pack is removed, and the nurse must keep the area free from oozing blood and excess saliva (using a supply of cotton wool rolls and pledgets to apply pressure).*
- *if there is a change of archwire, the new size must be chosen and prepared (the existing archwire may be reused).*
- *the colour of O-rings is selected by the patient and prepared by the nurse.*
- these are put on using:
  - Mathieu pliers, which can hold O-rings, twist ligatures, place elastics or chain
  - Coon's pliers, which tie ligatures (not Quickligs)
  - Twirl-ons, a hand instrument which stretches O-rings open to place over the tie wings of a bracket
  - Haemostats, which holds O-rings, ties ligatures and Quickligs, and can place chain
  - mosquitos, which hold O-rings, tie ligatures and Quickligs, and can place chain.
- the O-rings on the fixed appliance are removed.
- the archwire is taken out and either adjusted or replaced.
- o-rings or ligatures are placed around each bracket (often tied in a figure-of-eight pattern that holds the archwire under increased tension in the bracket slot)
- traction is then applied to the exposed canine using elastic thread or power chain from the archwire.
- if spool elastic is used on the links of gold chain, it is fed into the bracket and manually wound round the wire, tied under tension and the excess cut off.
- care must be taken that the 'tied ends' are not sharp and digging into the lips.
- the archwire is checked that it is not too long distally.

- *the patient is given oral hygiene instructions and another appointment* (this is usually only a few weeks away as it is important to renew the traction in order to maintain a consistent and sustained tension).
- *the patient is shown what has been done and given dietary instructions.*

This process is repeated until the tooth has been drawn into the line of the arch. It is usually necessary to reposition the bracket on the exposed canine during the course of this treatment. The subsequent bracket needs to be bonded onto the buccal aspect to achieve full alignment of the tooth.

Buccally positioned canines

If the canine is lying buccally, then it is possible to use a removable appliance prior to a fixed appliance to start extrusion (vertical downward movement) on the upper buccal canine.

If the patient's treatment involves a removable appliance

The nurse needs to prepare:

- *the patient's clinical notes*
- *the patient's models*
- *mirror, probe and College tweezers*
- *Adam's pliers*
- *spring-forming pliers*
- *Mauns cutters*
- *ruler*
- *dividers*
- *disposable archwire markers*
- *sharps box.*

Chairside procedure

- *the nurse needs to ensure that the patient and staff wear personal protection.*
- *the nurse checks that the patient is seated comfortably in the chair.*
- the clinician checks that the wound is clear from debris.
- the removable appliance is tried in.
- the clasps are adjusted to give maximum retention.
- the whip arm is adjusted to fit over the top (gingival) aspect of the bracket.
- the end of this is shortened as necessary and cinched (i.e. turned back on itself) to avoid a sharp end damaging the soft tissue.
- the patient is instructed on how to take the appliance in and out of the mouth.
- the patient practices doing this.
- they are then shown how to position and place the whip arm.
- the whip arm is then activated.

ECTOPIC CANINES

- *the patient is given instructions on care of the appliance and oral hygiene.*
- *another appointment is arranged for a few weeks' time to reactivate the whip arm, in order to maintain continuous force on the tooth.*

The widespread popularity of fixed appliance therapy now makes it:

- the preferred method when drawing ectopic palatal and buccal canines into the correct positions
- essential if both left and right canines have to be exposed simultaneously and there are other features of a malocclusion that also have to be corrected
- most effective if they have to be moved heroic distances.

ECTOPIC CANINES

Chapter 17
Debonding

When the active phase of fixed appliance treatment is complete, the bonds and bands need to be removed. This process in known as 'debonding'. A long appointment should be scheduled for this much-welcomed and long-awaited procedure.

The appointment for the removal of the fixed appliance may be anything from 1 to 2 years after the start of treatment, longer if it forms part of multidisciplinary treatment. For teenage patients this represents a significant percentage of their lives. For them, and for the whole team, this appointment is eagerly anticipated!

Occasionally, one dental arch is treated before the other, e.g. if the bite needs to be opened. However, it is uncommon for two arches to be debonded on separate occasions and as a general rule both upper and lower appliances are removed at the same appointment.

Just as the fitting of the fixed appliance took longer than the average appointment, so the removal of the appliance needs more time too.

PREPARATION

The nurse will need to prepare the tray for debanding (Figure 17.1):

- *the patient's clinical notes*
- *the patient's model box*
- *anterior bracket-removing pliers (Figure 17.2)*
- *mouth mirror, probe and College tweezers*
- *anterior ceramic bracket-removing pliers if needed*
- *band-removing pliers (Figure 17.3)*
- *band-slitting pliers (Figure 17.4)*
- *Mitchell trimmer*
- *adhesive-removing pliers (Figure 17.5)*
- *contra-angled handpiece and debonding bur (Figure 17.6)*
- *prophylactic paste and rubber cup*
- *sharps container for wire, brackets, etc.*
- *3-in-1 syringe*

Basic Guide to Orthodontic Dental Nursing, Second Edition. Fiona Grist.
© 2020 John Wiley & Sons Ltd. Published 2020 by John Wiley & Sons Ltd.

DEBONDING

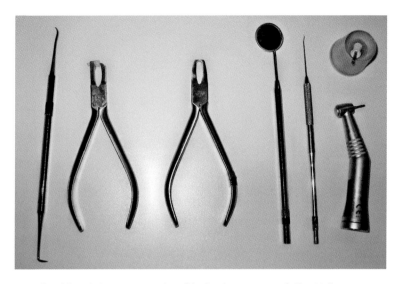

Figure 17.1 Tray for deband. Source: Reproduced by kind permission of Alan Hall.

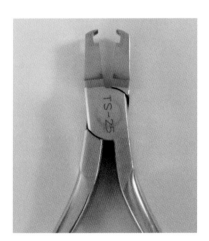

Figure 17.2 Anterior bracket-removing pliers. Source: Reproduced by kind permission of Alan Hall.

- *suction*
- *floss*
- *hand mirror*
- *alginate, bowl and spatula*
- *upper and lower impression trays*
- *wax knife and wax for bite*
- *method of softening wax (blowtorch, hot water, etc.)*
- *impression disinfectant solution, bag for impressions in transit*
- *laboratory form (to go with impressions to the technician)*
- *camera and lip retractors (if photographic records are needed)*
- *X-ray request form (if end of treatment radiographs are needed at this appointment).*

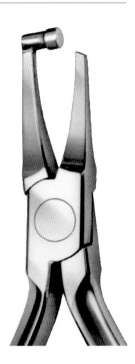

Figure 17.3 Band-removing pliers. Source: Reproduced by kind permission of Ortho-Care (UK) Ltd.

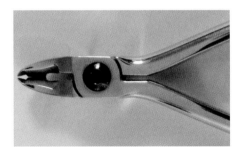

Figure 17.4 Band-slitting pliers. Source: Reproduced by kind permission of Alan Hall.

PROCEDURE

- *the nurse ensures that the patient and staff wear personal protection (it is vital that protective tinted glasses are worn for this procedure).*
- *the patient is made comfortable in the chair.*
- bands are then loosened and subsequently removed from molar teeth along with any residual cement.
- some clinicians remove O-rings or ligatures from around the metal brackets, others take it off in one piece (Figure 17.7).
- archwire is removed and then brackets are removed.
- some clinicians remove metal brackets and archwire together.
- archwire is often removed from brackets prior to removal of ceramic brackets (non-metal brackets such as ceramic ones are often more difficult to remove and can shatter in the process. It is vital that adequate eye protection is worn for this procedure).

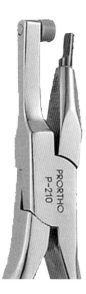

Figure 17.5 Adhesive-removing pliers. Source: Reproduced by kind permission of Ortho-Care (UK) Ltd.

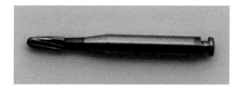

Figure 17.6 Debonding bur. Source: Reproduced by kind permission of Alan Hall.

- any remaining adherent cement is removed from the molars using a Mitchell trimmer.
- if buccal tubes have been used instead of bands, they are removed.
- any residual adhesive left after the buccal tubes or brackets have been taken off is removed. (This is done using a slow contra-angled handpiece and a debonding bur which removes adhesive but does not damage the enamel. Burs can be fine, coarse, rose-head or tapered.)
- floss is used between contact points.
- thorough polishing is performed using a contra-angled handpiece, rubber cup and prophylactic paste.

If a fixed retainer is to be fitted, it can be:

- previously fabricated by the technician
- bespoke, made by the clinician at the time
- a commercially made one.

It is fitted using the same method as that used to fit brackets.

- upper and lower alginate impressions and wax squash bite are taken.
- impressions and bite are disinfected before going to the laboratory.
- laboratory form is filled in requesting:
  - study models
  - upper retainer, usually Hawley or Essix (including the design for a Hawley)
  - lower retainer, usually Essix.

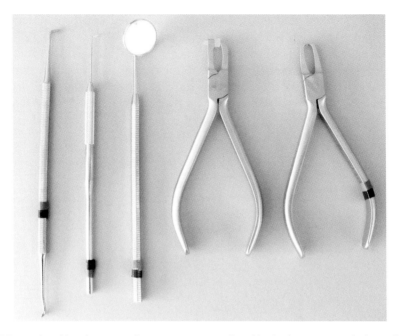

Figure 17.7 Band and bracket removal tray. Source: Reproduced by kind permission of Alan Hall.

Also, the pre- and post-treatment study models have to be filed in the patient's model box for quality control and clinical audit, or if digitally recorded entered onto the system. They can then be scored using Peer Assessment Rating (PAR) to measure how much improvement has been achieved by the orthodontic treatment.

A custom-made gum shield can now be organised if the patient plays contact sports. For the duration of the 'fixed appliance' period, the patient will have used a moldable gum shield as the position of the teeth changes so frequently.

To complete the existing photographic record, clinical photos are then taken, both intra- and extra-orally. End-of-treatment radiographs may also be taken at this appointment if clinically indicated.

After all traces of the appliance have been removed and the patient has had an opportunity to admire their teeth, there is a further discussion regarding oral hygiene.

For patients who have had the fixed appliances in place for 18 months to 2 years the teeth may be stained. This may be due to:

- tea and coffee
- red wine and tobacco
- curries
- all foods that have a high level of colouring.

After the deband appointment it may be necessary for the teeth to be professionally cleaned and polished. The hygienist will remove any calculus (a mixture of food, saliva and bacteria) that is present on the teeth around the gingival margins and areas that have been difficult to access.

Before fitting the fixed appliances, the teeth were cleaned with prophylactic paste that was oil-free. Now, paste that is slightly more abrasive is used.

After the appliance has been removed, patients are encouraged to spend some time flossing their teeth, paying special attention to their gums, before the next appointment when removable retainers are fitted and they start the retention stage of treatment. Often around this time some patients are keen to have their teeth whitened … but that is another conversation.

Chapter 18

Retention and retainers

In 1934 Albin Oppenheim, a medically and dentally qualified clinician said:

> "Retention is one of the most difficult problems in orthodontia, in fact, it is **the** problem."

This may be a statement that still holds true today: maintaining teeth in their corrected position remains challenging. The regime of wearing retainers in some form for the rest of the patient's life is now the gold standard of retention. Retention comes after the active treatment is completed when the appliance is removed. It is a passive stage and an important part of treatment. When it fails it is known as **relapse**.

After the end of active treatment and after deband, the surrounding tissues have yet to consolidate. Because teeth have been moved away from their original position, new alveolar bone has to form and consolidate and the gingival fibres have to adapt. The teeth need many months to 'firm up', so it is especially important to diligently wear retainers in the early stages. The patient must therefore understand that they need to wear the retainers to maintain good results or else everyone's hard work and effort will be undone.

What type of retention and for how long it is to be used is prescribed by the clinician and is part of the treatment plan. If the patient does not comply with the instructions and the teeth move some way out of alignment, returning to fixed appliances is often the only way of retrieving the situation. However, the patient may have run out of compliance and, in the NHS funded service, retreatment is rarely offered.

However, there can be other reasons for results to relapse.

- there can be unfavourable growth, often in the mandible.
- teeth do not fully intercuspate or interdigitate (fit together) in occlusion so that there is scope for them to slip out of position.

Two terms are used to describe how the teeth 'fit' together:

- intercuspate (the correct and preferred term)
- interdigitate.

When the teeth are in occlusion, they 'mesh' (intercuspate), like closing your hands together and putting your fingers (digits) between one another (hence the term interdigitate).

Basic Guide to Orthodontic Dental Nursing, Second Edition. Fiona Grist.
© 2020 John Wiley & Sons Ltd. Published 2020 by John Wiley & Sons Ltd.

Retainers can be:

- a removable type
- fixed to the teeth.

There are no standard criteria for the length of time you need to wear a retainer, and a longer retention period may be needed depending on the complexity of movement achieved. For removable retainers, some clinicians used to advise:

- full time for a year
- then 6 months, night-time only
- then discontinue.

Others advised full time for a year, then nights only for 6 months, then reduce the wear down to a couple of nights a week.

However, the current advice is that the frequency and time for which a retainer is worn can be reduced but **never** discontinued. It may be worn for only a couple of nights a week but this is still vital. If for any reason the retainer should suddenly feel tight, it should be worn more regularly for a little while until the tightness stops. This means that wearing retainers indefinitely on this occasional basis will be for life.

It is important to fit the retainers as soon as possible after active treatment has finished and the fixed appliances have been removed.

REMOVABLE RETAINERS

The most common forms are:

- Hawley retainers
- Essix retainers
- occasionally, removable appliances that have been made passive.

Hawley retainers

These consist of:

- an acrylic baseplate which fits around the palatal upper and lingual lower gum margins for stability
- metal clasps and rests
- a labial bow which fits over the front of the anterior teeth
- Adams cribs, usually positioned on the first molars for retention (Figures 18.1 and 18.2).

Begg retainers

These consist of:

- an acrylic baseplate
- a labial bow from the upper second molars with U-loops on the first molars
- no Adams cribs on the molars (Figure 18.3).

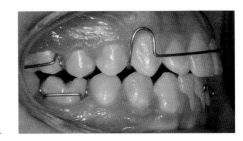

Figure 18.1 Labial bow and Adams crib. Source: Reproduced by kind permission of Jonathan Sandler.

(a)   (b)

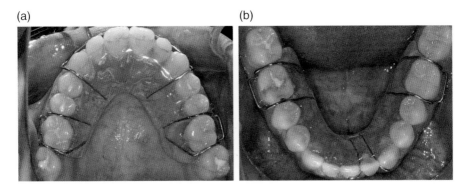

Figure 18.2 (a) Upper and (b) lower Hawley retainer. Source: Reproduced by kind permission of Jonathan Sandler.

Both these retainers are:

- worn full time
- worn when eating
- removed for cleaning
- removed and replaced by a gum shield for contact sports
- are quite discreet, as only a thin wire is visible.

Barrer spring appliance

This is an active retainer and is used to align marginally irregular incisors and then to retain them in that position. It is designed on a sectional working model on which the teeth have been repositioned in ideal alignment and applies force both lingually and buccally. Interproximal reduction may be used. To avoid the risk of inhalation, some later versions include distal extensions of acrylic (Figure 18.4).

Essix retainers

An Essix retainer:

- is a light, clear, 'gum shield'-type appliance
- does not have any wires
- is a vacuum-formed appliance made from thermoplastic material.

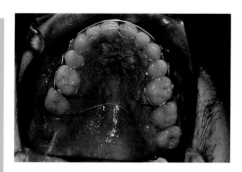

Figure 18.3 Begg retainer. Source: Reproduced by kind permission of Jonathan Sandler.

(a)   (b)

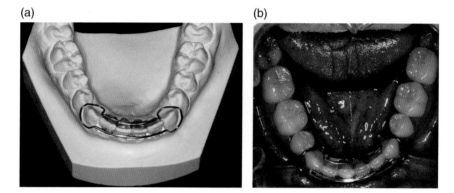

Figure 18.4 (a) Original design of a Barrer spring appliance. Source: Reproduced by kind permission of Simon Littlewood. (b) A Barrer appliance in situ. Source: Reproduced by kind permission of Jonathan Sandler.

These are:

- lighter
- less visible
- not worn for eating and drinking
- often worn just at night.

Essix retainers (Figure 18.5) are sometimes used in the lower arch if:

- it might be hard to get good retention using a Hawley type
- the patient would tolerate it better
- an adult patient would find it socially more acceptable.

Positioners

Positioners are sometimes fitted at the end of treatment.

- these are flexible splints which are mildly active.
- they continue to correct any small or mild irregularities which still remain after the active appliances have been removed.

These devices are made by the technician to a very exact prescription.

RETENTION AND RETAINERS

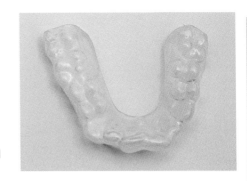

Figure 18.5 Essix retainer. Source: Reproduced by kind permission of Alan Hall.

Making removable retainers

For making a removable Hawley or Essix retainer at deband, in addition to the debanding instruments the nurse will need to prepare:

- *upper and lower impressions*
- *a wax bite*
- *wax knife and method of softening the wax*
- *disinfectant solution for the impressions and bite*
- *a laboratory instruction sheet.*

At the fitting of a removable Hawley or Essix retainer, the nurse needs to prepare:

- *the patient's clinical notes*
- *the patient's model box*
- *the retainer/retainers from the laboratory*
- *mirror, probe and College tweezers*
- *a protective retainer case for the patient to use when the retainer is not being worn (e.g. contact sports)*
- *instruction leaflet*
- *a hand mirror.*

plus for a Hawley retainer:

- *Adams pliers (Figure 18.6)*
- *spring-forming pliers*
- *straight handpiece and acrylic bur for adjustments to the acrylic.*

Procedure

- *the nurse ensures that the patient and staff wear personal protection.*
- *the nurse makes sure that the patient is comfortable.*
- the retainer is fitted in the mouth.
- a check is made that it fits well and is comfortable.
- any adjustment is then made.
- the patient is shown how to remove it.
- the patient is shown how to insert it.
- *instruction is given on when to wear it, how to clean it and oral hygiene.*

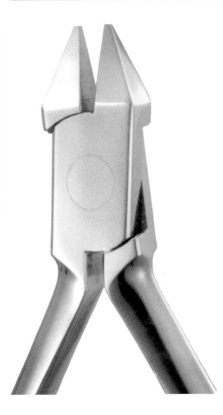

Figure 18.6 Adams pliers. Source: Reproduced by kind permission of Ortho-Care (UK) Ltd.

- *an instruction leaflet is also given.*
- *the patient is given a protective case.*
- *the Medical Devices form is filed in the patient's notes.*

For safety, the retainers need to be kept in a firm container when not being worn (Figure 18.7).

FIXED RETAINERS

Fixed retainers consist of a fine multi-flex wire or similar flexible length of metal attachment, which is bonded directly onto the lingual or palatal surface of the anterior teeth and which keeps them in position and joined together. They can be used in addition to Essix retainers, which are fitted over the fixed retainer.

This is often used when:

- extra retention is needed
- there is a possibility that midline spacing (diastemas) may open (Figure 18.8)
- when there has been correction of severely rotated teeth
- when the patient may not respond well to wearing a removable retainer adequately
- where the occlusal intercuspation may contribute to instability.

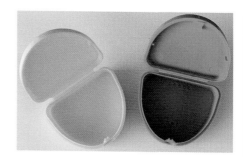

Figure 18.7 Retainer cases. Source: Reproduced by kind permission of Ortho-Care (UK) Ltd.

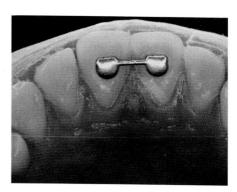

Figure 18.8 Fixed retainer to prevent diastema reopening. Source: Reproduced by kind permission of Alan Hall.

The fixed retainer (Figure 18.9):

- is not visible, placed on the lingual or palatal surfaces of the teeth
- is small and discreet
- does not interfere with speech
- can be used in addition to a removable retainer
- is not uncomfortable to the tongue
- gives patients peace of mind.

However:

- it does need to be regularly checked by the clinician
- because it is harder to use floss where there is a permanent wire, special efforts must be made with oral hygiene in those areas
- because the adhesives used are similar to those for a fixed appliance, the patient has to avoid the same foods and drinks that may be harmful, e.g. hard, sticky, crunchy or acidic

Fitting a fixed (bonded) retainer

The fixed retainer is normally fitted at the deband appointment.

- there are wires commercially available that can be used from the spool and fixed into place (Figure 18.10).
- some wire-fixed retainers can be made in the laboratory by the technician. For this, an impression or scan is taken for a work model on the last adjustment appointment. The technician fabricates the wire on this model.

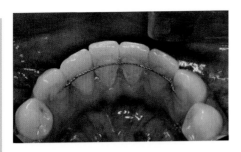

Figure 18.9 Fixed retainer. Source: Reproduced by kind permission of Jonathan Sandler.

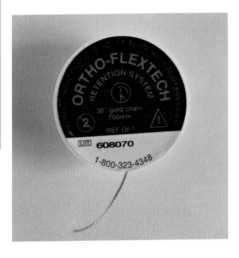

Figure 18.10 Wire for fixed retainers. Source: Reproduced by kind permission of Ortho-Care (UK) Ltd.

Multi-strand wire gives flexibility for this as does flexible gold link chain. The fixed palatal retainer must not interfere with the bite of the teeth on closing.

At the deband appointment:

- the upper and lower fixed appliances, i.e. all brackets, bands, tubes, cleats, etc., are removed
- all residual adhesive and cement is cleaned off
- the teeth are cleaned with an oil-free prophylactic paste
- the fixed retainer is then bonded in place
- upper and lower alginate impressions are taken
- a wax squash bite (to record the occlusion) is taken
- these are disinfected prior to going to the laboratory.

The nurse will need to prepare:

- *the patient's models*
- *the model and retainer from the laboratory if relevant*
- *contra-angled handpiece, composite finishing burs*
- *disposable Dappen's pots*
- *etchant and primer or self-etch primer*
- *adhesive, ones specifically for lingual retainers*
- *mirror, probe and College tweezers*
- *floss*

- *LED light*
- *the wire for the retainer that the clinician requests or prefers*
- *3-in-1 syringe*
- *aspirator*
- *saliva ejectors*
- *cheek retractors*
- *cotton wool rolls*
- *prophylaxis handpiece, rubber cup and paste*
- *hand scaling instruments*
- *special protective glasses for clinician, patient and nurse*
- *Weingart pliers*

(a)   (b)

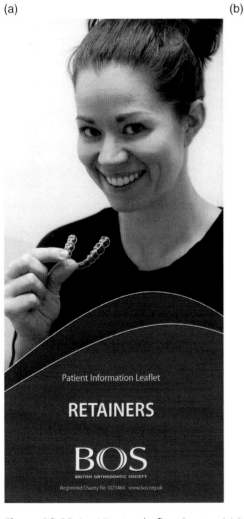

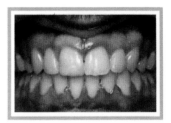

Now your teeth
are straight...

keep them
that way!

Figure 18.11 (a–c) Retainer leaflets. Sources: (a) Reproduced by kind permission of British Orthodontic Society. (b, c) Reproduced by kind permission of Ortho-Care (UK) Ltd.

(c)

Retention: a reasoned approach.

Follow your Orthodontist's instructions carefully, because the advice will be based on your own particular needs. However, nobody knows for sure how much retainers really need to be worn, because each case is different. You could try this approach:

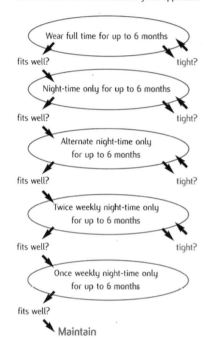

Wear full time for up to 6 months

fits well?   tight?

Night-time only for up to 6 months

fits well?   tight?

Alternate night-time only for up to 6 months

fits well?   tight?

Twice weekly night-time only for up to 6 months

fits well?   tight?

Once weekly night-time only for up to 6 months

fits well?

Maintain

Remember

To keep your teeth straight you will need to wear your retainers on an intermittent night only basis indefinitely.

If your retainers no longer fit, it is because you have not worn them enough.

Keep your retainers clean or they will start to smell!

Keep your retainers safe by always storing them in your retainer box.

Even with good retainer wear a little movement is to be expected following treatment.

Clean your retainers in a proprietary brand of disinfectant solution on a daily basis.

You have expensive teeth - look after them!

© Ortho-Care (UK) Ltd 2017

Figure 18.11 *(Continued)*

- *light wire cutters*
- *light wire pliers*
- *flat plastic.*

Procedure

- *the nurse ensures the patient and staff wear personal protection.*
- *the patient is made comfortable.*
- after the upper and lower fixed appliances have been removed, the teeth are cleaned using rubber cup and prophylaxis paste after using scalers (mostly in adult patients) to remove any deposits of calculus.
- cheek retractors, saliva ejectors and cotton rolls, etc. are put in to maintain a dry field.

- the wire previously made on the model is tried in, or wire or gold chain is then cut and customised to fit exactly and is tried in.
- the area is etched, washed and redried.
- the area is primed or self-etch primer applied.
- adhesive is applied to lingual surface of each tooth to be included in the bonding process.
- the wire is seated into the adhesive on the teeth.
- some clinicians use floss to stabilise the wire.
- adhesive is cured with LED light.
- any further adhesive that is required is added.
- added adhesive is cured.
- the retainer is checked to ensure it is not rough to the tongue and soft tissues.
- if the patient is also to have an Essix retainer:
  - take upper and lower impressions
  - take wax squash bite to record the occlusion.
- the patient is given instructions on how to maintain the retainer.
- the patient is given leaflets (Figure 18.11) and an appointment to check the fixed retainer in the future.

Chapter 19

Aligners

When this book was first published, the chapter on aligners began with the sentence:

> In addition to the conventional systems of removable and fixed appliances, there are now methods of straightening and de-rotating overcrowded teeth by using aligners.

It would not be an exaggeration to say that in recent years their development and scope has been stellar. What was true then is certainly not now. Effective marketing means the public has become much more aware of them, fueling demand for this treatment. Furthermore, the range of malocclusion that can be treated has greatly expanded.

Aligner treatment comprises a series of removable aligners often designed by a computer software package and used in sequence by the patient.

Advantages to the patient

- less visible than labial fixed appliances
- less costly than lingual fixed appliances
- easily removed for eating, drinking (other than still water), cleaning and special occasions.

Advantages to the clinician

- require less chairside time
- fewer appointments
- emergencies are less likely.

Disadvantages

- an aligner must be worn for sufficient time to achieve tooth movement.
- loss or damage to an aligner causes delay and further cost.
- in order to achieve three-dimensional tooth movements (e.g. torque), attachments may need to be bonded to teeth that make the aligners less aesthetic; this can be traumatic to lips and cheeks, in a similar fashion to fixed brace attachments.

Basic Guide to Orthodontic Dental Nursing, Second Edition. Fiona Grist.
© 2020 John Wiley & Sons Ltd. Published 2020 by John Wiley & Sons Ltd.

TYPES OF ALIGNERS

There are two types of aligner treatment.

- type 1: a single appliance that is adjusted by the clinician.
- type 2: a series of computer-generated aligners.

Type 1

This, the first type of aligner treatment, is marketed by Intelligent Alignment Systems (IAS) and uses a single appliance, the Inman Aligner®.

Unlike the other system, this appliance:

- has moveable parts
- uses a piston such as NiTi coil springs
- has labial and lingual components.

The appliance consists of a baseplate and moving parts. The lingual coil springs put controlled pressure on the lingual aspects of teeth while an acrylic-coated stainless steel labial bar exerts an opposing pressure. This dual pressure squeezes the teeth so that they are eased into alignment. Patients are instructed to wear the aligner for 20 hours a day, with the duration of treatment being between 6 and 16 weeks. This type of appliance is not as discreet as clear aligners.

Initial appointment

To begin this treatment, the nurse needs to prepare:

- *the patient's model box*
- *upper and lower impression trays*
- *silicone putty impression material and bite registration paste*
- *disinfectant solution for impressions and bite*
- *bag and laboratory instructions*
- *form for instructions for the technician.*

Procedure

- *the nurse ensures that the patient and staff wear personal protection.*
- *the nurse makes sure that the patient is sitting comfortably.*
- upper and lower impressions for study and work models are taken.
- bite registration is recorded.
- *the impressions and bite are disinfected and bagged and sent to the technician.*
- *the nurse ensures that the laboratory sheet is completed.*
- intra- and extra-oral photographs are taken.
- *the patient is given instructions on the new appliance and is told what to expect at the next visit.*

Fitting appointment

When the patient returns for the fitting appointment, the nurse needs to prepare:

- *the aligner to be fitted*
- *the patient's model box*
- *mouth mirror*
- *ruler*
- *Adams pliers*
- *interproximal reduction kit if required*
- *oscillating handpiece and shaped burs*
- *handpiece and acrylic bur*
- *hand mirror*
- *patient instruction leaflets.*

Procedure

- *the nurse needs to ensure that the patient and staff wear personal protection.*
- *the nurse makes sure that the patient is sitting comfortably.*
- *the work from the laboratory is made ready.*
- a stripping kit or oscillating handpiece is used as required.
- the aligner is fitted.
- aligner is trimmed with acrylic bur if necessary.
- Adams pliers are used to adjust the appliance as necessary.
- ruler is used to record spaces and rotations.
- *the patient is given instruction on how to remove and insert the appliances.*
- *the patient is given an instruction leaflet on cleaning and care of the appliances.*

The patient must be seen at regular intervals.

When the required alignment has been achieved, the patient must have impressions taken for:

- retainers
- end-of-treatment study models.

As with all appliances and aligners made in a laboratory, they must have a Medical Devices certificate issued when they are made. This records:

- the materials used and their properties
- their batch numbers
- details of who made the appliances.

This certificate must always be filed in the patient's notes after fitting any appliance.

Retention

This can comprise a new 'conventional' retainer or the original Inman Aligner modified to be passive.

Type 2

These aligners (Figure 19.1) are:

- made to be worn sequentially
- manufactured to fit the crowns of teeth, like Essix retainers
- made of polyester or thermoplastic polyurethane
- suitable for both adults and children
- manufactured by certified providers.

They must be:

- worn for 22 hours every day
- upgraded approximately every 1–2 weeks
- reviewed by the clinician every 4–6 weeks.

The computer-aided design/computer-aided manufacturing (CAD/CAM) software for predicting the tooth movement needed to correct a malocclusion was developed by Align Technology in the 1990s. While other companies have developed similar systems, the original system, Invisalign®, still has the biggest market share.

Whilst initial aligners could merely tip the crowns of teeth in non-extraction cases, they can now:

- produce crown movements, such as de-rotation and extrusion, by the clinician adding composite 'attachments' as directed by the prescription
- add computer-generated ridges within the aligners that, combined with buccal attachments, produce root movements
- act as functional appliances by adapting the occlusal surfaces
- use fixed intra-oral anchorage points (e.g. temporary anchorage devices, TADs) for use with inter-arch elastics
- be used for extraction cases and complex malocclusions.

Initial appointment

On completion of the initial assessment and when a treatment plan is formulated, the following clinical records are taken:

- intra and extra-oral photographs
- radiographs
- silicone impressions and a bite registration or three-dimensional scan of the dentition.

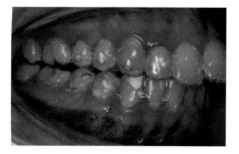

Figure 19.1 Patient wearing upper and lower clear aligners. Source: Reproduced by kind permission of Jonathan Sandler.

The nurse needs to prepare:

- *silicone impression putty and bite registration paste*
- *upper and lower impressions trays (or record a three-dimensional scan)*
- *plastic bag for completed documents and impressions*
- *camera*
- *cheek retractors*
- *mouth mirror.*

Procedure

- *the nurse ensures that the patient and staff wear personal protection.*
- *the patient is made comfortable.*
- *nurse takes or assists in taking impressions and bite recording.*
- *the impressions and bite registration are disinfected and bagged.*
- *the laboratory sheet is completed.*
- *the nurse takes/or assists in taking intra- and extra-oral photographs.*
- *check the patient's consent has been obtained for transfer of records and personal data to aligner manufacturer.*
- *the patient is given instruction leaflet and information on forthcoming treatment.*

The impression and bite registrations are all sent to the laboratory with a detailed treatment and instruction plan. Three-dimensional scans are sent electronically along with digital copies of photographs and radiographs.

Using computer software, the technicians will then:

- create a model of the desired finished result
- calculate the required movement each aligner must be programmed with to achieve this
- calculate the number of aligners that will be needed
- calculate how much interproximal stripping is needed (if it is needed).

The manufacturer will send back an electronic prediction of how the teeth will be moved. Requests for modifications can be made until the clinician is satisfied that the measurements for a series of aligners to move the teeth into the positions on the generated model are complete. The calculations are then transferred to their laboratory where the aligners are manufactured.

A series of aligners is then made that are:

- bespoke
- graded
- to be used in sequence
- all made at the same time
- sent back to the clinician
- also able be used as bleaching trays.

Each aligner will move the teeth an exact amount.

Fitting the aligner

Before the patient arrives, the nurse needs to:

- *check that aligners and documentation matches the patient*
- *check whether attachments are to be fitted on this appointment.*

If this is the case, the nurse must prepare:

- *medium-density, flowable enamel-coloured composite*
- *bonding agent (if bonding to porcelain, then a porcelain bonding agent is needed)*
- *acid etchant*
- *high- and low-volume suction and triple spray ends*
- *moisture control.*

Procedure

- *the nurse ensures that the patient and staff wear personal protection.*
- *the nurse makes the patient comfortable.*
- *the sites where buccal attachments are to be placed are checked.*
- the clinician will then isolate one arch, etch the appropriate buccal surfaces, apply bonding agent to etched enamel and light cure.
- *the nurse then fills the buccal extrusions in the separate attachment template which has been supplied by the manufacturer with composite, and hands to the clinician.*
- the clinician then seats this onto the dentition and light cures the composite.
- the soft plastic template is then peeled off, leaving the attachments on the teeth.
- the same procedure is repeated for the other arch.

Some treatments involve interproximal reduction. This is a process outlined in the next section. Interproximal adjustment (if needed) has to be precise, as prescribed. The teeth are then moved into this space. The patient returns to the surgery at regular intervals to check and monitor progress.

The clinician fits the first set of aligners and explains to the patient how to insert and remove them.

The nurse needs to prepare:

- *hand-held mirror*
- *leaflets on wear and how to look after them*
- *chewies® (small foam cylinders for the patient to bite on to seat the aligner)*
- *the box to store the aligner when not in the mouth (supplied by the manufacturer).*

Initially, the aligners feel tight but this eases as the teeth move. Patients are given two or three sets of aligners and advised to upgrade to the next set after about 2 weeks. There are regular checks on progress, and for interproximal reduction, as necessary until the last set of aligners has achieved the final result.

Retention

As with all tooth movement, there must be a period of consolidation to prevent relapse. Many manufacturers use additionally strengthened aligners to act as retainers and some clinicians opt for fixed retainers too. End-of-treatment records must be now taken.

ALIGNERS

INTERPROXIMAL REDUCTION

Sometimes it is necessary to create space in order to move crowded teeth into a better position. The method for gaining a small amount of space is called interproximal reduction (also known as interproximal stripping and interdental enamel reduction). The method can provide up to 8 mm of space per arch spread over a number of teeth (Figure 19.2).

This technique can also be used selectively in fixed appliance therapy in the following circumstances:

- where it is necessary to de-rotate a single tooth
- if there is an area of very mild localised crowding
- to eliminate dark triangles
- to improve the shape of the papilla
- when re-shaping and contouring (Figure 19.3).

Stripping or slenderising removes tiny amounts of proximal enamel from:

- either the mesial or distal contact point (or both) of the tooth
- the adjacent tooth if more appropriate.

This provides space for the tooth to be moved into alignment.
Interproximal reduction can be done either:

- manually, or
- using an air rotor.

The handpiece method is becoming more widespread because:

- it is easier to use at the back of the mouth
- the oscillating movement causes less striation of the enamel
- it is less likely to cause periodontal damage.

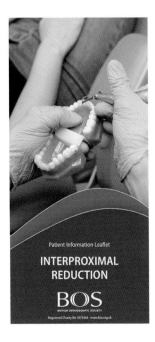

Figure 19.2 British Orthodontic Society interproximal reduction leaflet.
Source: Reproduced by kind permission of the British Orthodontic Society.

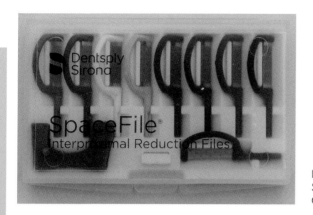

Figure 19.3 Interproximal reduction kit. Source: Reproduced by kind permission of Ortho-Care (UK) Ltd.

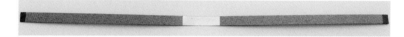

Figure 19.4 Interproximal strip. Source: Reproduced by kind permission of Ortho-Care (UK) Ltd.

Air rotor

This method is usually used on adult patients. In the use of an air rotor, the following tools (carbide or diamond) are used:

- cutting discs
- contouring discs
- cutting burs
- finishing burs.

When discs are used, a guard must be in place to protect the patient's soft tissues. Up to 8 mm, spread amongst several teeth, can be gained in an arch. This technique does not cause such striations on the enamel surface as the manual method.

Manually

This method is:

- slower
- uses a sawing action
- may be easier when monitoring the amount of enamel to be removed
- used an interproximal strip (Figure 19.4).

The interproximal strips:

- are single use
- made of stainless steel, often diamond-coated
- are of varying thickness
- have a fine or coarse texture
- are either single or double sided
- can be saw or serrated strips.

There is an anterior instrument and a posterior instrument. The posterior instrument works on teeth at the back of the mouth where access may be difficult, so is angled to give greater ease of working.

A number of instruments are available which are designed to accurately measure the amount of space that needs to be achieved before and after stripping. These include:

- incremental thickness gauges (a set of graded stainless-steel gauges, like small rulers, that fit between the teeth after stripping to measure the gap)
- an interdental measurement gauge (a hand-held instrument with a cylindrical end that, when inserted into the gaps, calculates how much space has been created).

Patients may experience temporary dental sensitivity following interproximal reduction. To minimise this, they are asked to use fluoride gel (easily applied using a manual tooth-brush) to help with re-mineralisation of the enamel. This gel is similar to that used by patients:

- with decalcification
- who have had a course of tooth whitening.

ALIGNERS

Chapter 20

Multi-disciplinary orthodontics

For dental patients, orthodontic treatment is often part of a multidisciplinary team approach. These patients fall into three main categories of combined need:

- restorative
- surgical
- cleft.

Some patients, for example those with a cleft condition, may require treatment in all three categories.

RESTORATIVE

Some simple cases are multidisciplinary involving the general dental practitioner (GDP) and the orthodontist but more severe cases are seen for a full assessment on an orthodontic/restorative/surgical multidisciplinary clinic.

Microdontia (small teeth)

These patients sometimes have conical or 'spiky' teeth. The most common tooth affected is the upper lateral incisor. These teeth are often referred to as peg-shaped laterals. These irregularly shaped teeth may have to be built up with composite facings, veneers or crowns to achieve the best aesthetic result. Sometimes several teeth are affected.

Hypodontia (congenitally missing teeth)

These patients do not have all the teeth needed to make up the full dentition. Rarely, they can have both the deciduous and permanent tooth missing. If this is just a single tooth, it may be possible to close the space orthodontically using braces. If the span is too wide, then it is necessary to use some type of replacement. This could be:

- a bridge
- an implant.

Basic Guide to Orthodontic Dental Nursing, Second Edition. Fiona Grist.
© 2020 John Wiley & Sons Ltd. Published 2020 by John Wiley & Sons Ltd.

Some patients with hypodontia have several missing teeth, even three or more per quadrant. Orthodontic treatment can be invaluable in correcting the existing permanent teeth into position to facilitate the restoration of spaces left by the absence of a number of teeth.

Often hypodontia and microdontia are found in the same patient.

SURGICAL

Some patients are born with, or develop later in life:

- facial deformity
- skeletal pattern imbalance
- problems with mandibular condyles
- unfavourable growth, especially in the mandible.

These may need corrective jaw surgery.

It may also be necessary to have surgery on:

- ectopic teeth which need surgical uncovering and exposure
- teeth which need transplanting to a more favourable position
- a thick fleshy frenum
- supernumerary, submerged or impacted teeth.

A close working relationship between the orthodontist and the maxillofacial surgery team is needed when the patient requires an osteotomy. This is a procedure to correct a skeletal discrepancy of mandible/maxilla. Patients are seen on a combined clinic, with both the orthodontists and maxillofacial surgeons present, when patients are given information and also leaflets (Figure 20.1).

Most osteotomies are carried out using incisions made inside the mouth. Sometimes bone is harvested from another site, often the hip (the iliac crest), for use in the procedure.

These procedures are carried out after the patient has finished most of their growth. In the case of the face, this is later for boys than girls.

Osteotomies can be:

- maxillary
- mandibular
- both (known as bimaxillary).

The maxillary (midface) osteotomies include:

- Le Fort I (involving the tooth-bearing maxilla)
- Le Fort II (involving the maxilla and the nose)
- Le Fort III (involving the maxilla, nose and cheeks).

The mandibular (lower face) osteotomies include:

- sagittal split (centred at the angles and ascending ramus of the mandible)
- genioplasty (when the tip of the chin is repositioned).

MULTI-DISCIPLINARY ORTHODONTICS

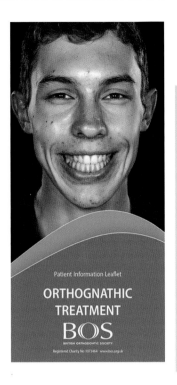

Figure 20.1 Leaflet for orthognathic surgery. Source: Reproduced by kind permission of the British Orthodontic Society.

For many patients these operations will alter their appearance. This is one of the reasons the patient may be offered an appointment with a clinical psychologist at this stage.

For these patients the orthodontist and maxillofacial surgeon together need to see patients to formulate a treatment plan. As part of this the orthodontist will take radiographs, including a lateral and occasionally a postero-anterior cephalogram on which to reproduce a tracing. This is now often done using computer software.

There are many reference points on a tracing for which skeletal measurements need to be recorded:

- horizontally, antero-posterior (front to back) length
- transversely, width across (less commonly used).

For the purposes of a basic guide, it would be useful as a baseline to see the following.

- Frankfort plane (Figure 20.2): as the horizontal measurement.
- maxillary plane: as a line from the posterior border to the anterior point of the hard palate.
- occlusal plane: as a line between the teeth in occlusion.
- mandibular plane: as the lower border of the mandible.
- aesthetic plane: as a line along the soft tissue profile from the tip of the nose to the tip of the chin.

Tracing can be done either manually (now less used) or using computer software. In order to make a manual tracing, the operator will need:

- tracing film, usually 8 × 10 inches (20 × 25 cm)
- a tooth-tracing template

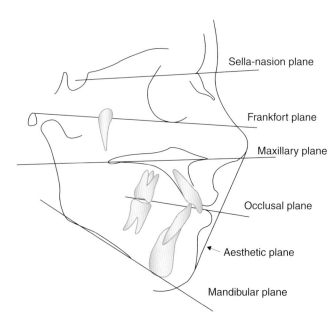

Figure 20.2 Drawing showing Frankfort plane. Source: Reproduced by kind permission of Alan Hall.

- triangle
- cephalometric protractor and template (joined)
- metric scale rule
- yellow graph pencil
- a light box.

The operator will:

- manually place the lateral cephalometric radiograph on the light box (with the nose facing to the right)
- place the tracing paper over this
- then using a series of recognised hard tissue coordinate points, trace lines between these points and measure the relevant angles
- using a tooth template, protractor and pencil produce a tracing that will accurately show the pre-surgical measurements of the patient and this helps form the proposed orthodontic and surgical planning.

NB Soft tissue profiles are not so predictable, but as a guide follow the bone changes by 50%.

When using a computer, the operator needs to trace the reference points which are plotted by the software program. This calculates the angles and measurements that, when printed out, are shown together with line tracings.

Orthodontic treatment will then be planned and carried out by putting the teeth in the positions they need to be in prior to the surgery. This can be done digitally or using traditional methods. At this stage, the laboratory technician may also be asked to make a Kesling set-up. This is done by taking a set of work models and cutting off and 'resetting' the teeth in their projected position. This can also be done using digitally enhanced models.

The aim of the procedure is to align the dental arches so they are coordinated and fit together at operation. This makes the post-surgical orthodontic stage simpler and shorter.

When initial records have been taken and the treatment plan has been agreed and finalised, the patient then has the treatment required to get the teeth into the correct preoperative position.

Pre-surgical orthodontics

For the nurse, these appointments need the same preparation as for a routine fixed appliance.

When the orthodontist is satisfied that the teeth are in the planned position prior to surgery, impressions are taken.

Co-ordination impressions

- are usually taken with the archwires in the mouth
- are of upper and lower alginate
- have a wax squash bite.

These impressions are cast by the technician. The co-ordination models are then checked by the orthodontist to ensure that the positioning of the teeth is correct and the proposed occlusion is correct for the planned surgical procedure.

At this stage, if the positioning and proposed occlusion are correct, an operation date is then arranged with the surgeon after they have reviewed the patient.

Co-ordination and communication is essential: all appointments between the two specialties, the laboratory and the patient have to be co-ordinated.

Countdown to surgery

With the co-ordination impressions completed and an appointment date booked for surgery, an appointment is made for further impressions a few weeks before the operation date. These are known as **wafer impressions**.

For this appointment the nurse needs to prepare:

- *the patient's model box*
- *a fixed appliance tray*
- *mirror, probe and College tweezers*
- *distal end pliers*
- *light wire pliers*
- *Weingart pliers*
- *crimping pliers for surgical hook placement*
- *ligatures*
- *Kobayashi ligatures*
- *Mathieu/mosquito pliers*
- *ligature director*
- *ligature tucker*
- *alginate, bowls and spatula*
- *upper and lower impression trays*

MULTI-DISCIPLINARY ORTHODONTICS

- *wax for bite registration*
- *solution to disinfect the impressions and bite*
- *equipment for taking facebow reading if necessary*
- *sharps box*
- *clinical camera*
- *photographic mirrors*
- *lip retractors*
- *patient relief wax.*

Chairside procedure

- the archwires are removed from both the maxilla and mandible.
- upper and lower alginate impressions are taken for the wafer, the planning models and orthodontic study models.
- a bite registration is taken.
- if the archwires have been removed, they are then 'tied in' (for strength, metal ligatures and crimpable hooks may be used to hold the archwires securely in the brackets).
- it is important that the appliance is robust and remains intact for the surgical operation and post-surgical orthodontic stage.
- intra- and extra-oral photographs are then taken.

NB If the patient is having a bimaxillary procedure, then a facebow measurement will also be taken.

The patient has now completed the pre-surgical phase of orthodontic treatment and is ready for the operation. The impressions and bite go to the laboratory where an acrylic wafer is made and model planning carried out in conjunction with the surgeon and orthodontist. This is to determine the correct occlusal position at operation.

This wafer will be used by the surgeon during the surgery. It is made of clear plastic and is placed between the teeth and used in theatre as a location guide for the occlusion.

Try-in of wafer

A week before the scheduled operation date, the wafer it 'tried in' to make sure that it fits correctly.

The operation

- most osteotomies are approached from inside the mouth.
- patients sometimes have external drains.
- the bony sections are normally held in position using titanium bone plates or screws.
- after surgery, patients may also be fitted with intermaxillary elastics to tightly hold the upper and lower dental arches in the planned post-operative position.
- how long the patient wears these depends on a number of factors and is decided by the maxillofacial surgeon and the orthodontist.

Post-operative appointment

After the operation the patient has an appointment with the orthodontist.

The nurse needs to prepare:

- *the patient's clinical notes*
- *radiographs*
- *the orthodontic planning box*
- *the surgical planning box*
- *a fixed appliance tray*
- *intermaxillary elastics*
- *hand mirror*
- *clinical camera*
- *photographic cheek retractors*
- *photographic mirrors.*

Chairside procedure

- *the dentist, nurse and patient wear personal protective equipment.*
- *the patient is made comfortable in the chair.*
- the occlusion is checked (the patient may still be swollen and sore).
- the clinician may wish to alter or reposition the pattern of elastics.
- cheeks and lips are checked for normal sensation (sometimes they have 'numb' or 'tingling' areas after the operation).
- *advice on oral hygiene and diet is given.*
- appropriate radiographs have usually been taken by the surgical team.

A further follow-up appointment is arranged with the patient.

The patient will continue to be bruised and to feel swollen for some while, but how much and for how long varies from patient to patient. This will eventually subside. However, the loss of feeling around the face, especially the lips and chin, may take longer to recede and for sensation to return to normal. Some patients notice tingling and feeling slowly returning up to a year after surgery and in some patients the sensation never returns to normal. Patients must take care not to bite or burn their lips when eating and drinking.

Patients will have been given advice about diet and oral hygiene. They will also be given instruction on how to change their elastics for the time that they are needed.

Post-surgical orthodontics

Usually, there is a period of post-surgical orthodontics to 'sock in' the bite and make sure that the bite fully intercuspates, which can last for 3–8 months. The patient is then ready for debanding of the fixed appliances and the fitting of retention appliances.

There is a protocol regarding when the patients are seen on combined clinics and where they are monitored and reviewed by the whole multidisciplinary team. The final review appointment is normally 2 years after debanding and further advice on retainer wear is given before discharge.

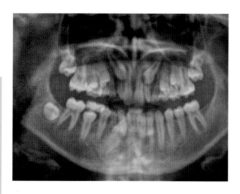

Figure 20.3 Radiograph of ectopic canines. Source:
Reproduced by kind permission of Jonathan Sandler.

Other surgical procedures undertaken in theatre

Sometimes patients need surgical extraction of:

- severely submerged teeth
- impacted teeth and buried supernumerary teeth.

The following may be undertaken under general anesthesia in theatre, or under local anesthesia.

- frenectomy: removal of frenum if implicated in a diastema or preventing space closure.
- removal of tongue tie: if causing serious clinical difficulties (see Chapter 1).

Uncovering ectopic canines

Patients can also have surgery to uncover unerupted ectopic canines (Figure 20.3). When these are exposed, a bracket or pad attached to a gold-plated chain is fitted on the tooth/teeth. Following the surgery, the patient will start treatment to apply traction to the chain from the fixed appliance and the process of drawing the canine into its correct position begins. As the distance shortens, the links of chain are reduced (see Chapter 16).

CLEFT LIP AND PALATE

As soon as they are born, babies born with a cleft of the lip and/or palate should be referred to the cleft team. Much of the specialist care of these babies is undertaken in hospital. They will also need routine dental check-ups with a GDP.

The cleft team may consist of:

- a cleft surgeon
- specialist cleft nurses
- an ear, nose and throat (ENT) surgeon
- a paediatric audiologist

MULTI-DISCIPLINARY ORTHODONTICS

- an orthodontist
- orthodontic nurses
- a paediatrician
- a paediatric dentist
- feeding advisors
- speech and language therapists (SALT)
- a geneticist.

The interface between these specialties provides the care pathway for these patients, which begins at birth and continues until they have completed their treatment, often in their late teens or early twenties.

Some parents are aware before delivery that their baby has a cleft, as this can be detected on foetal scans. For other parents the news comes as a complete shock. Cleft lip and palate is the most common congenital craniofacial deformity and affects all ethnic groups. Cleft surgeons come from a background of either maxillofacial or plastic surgery.

There are variations of clefting deformity, which is caused by abnormal facial development before birth. Clefts can also be a symptom of a syndrome or sequence, e.g. Pierre Robin sequence.

The word 'cleft' means a gap or fissure, where there has not been correct fusion between natural structures. This can manifest as:

- a cleft lip (cheiloschisis)
- a cleft palate (palatoschisis).

Some babies are born with both, with deformities ranging from a small notch in the upper lip to total bilateral cleft lip and alveolus extending to the hard and soft palates.

Patients can present with:

- cleft lip (unilateral or bilateral)
- cleft lip (unilateral or bilateral) plus hard and/or soft palate
- cleft palate only (hard and/or soft).

Clefts can involve:

- the maxillofacial skeleton
- soft tissue envelope
- the nasal structure
- the hard and soft palates
- the alveolar ridge
- the upper dental arch (Figure 20.4).

This cohort of patients will potentially undergo a series of operations and procedures over a period lasting from birth until they are in their late teens (Figures 20.6–20.9). They often have a lot to cope with apart from their teeth, such as:

- problems with feeding (as babies), necessitating the use of Haberman bottles and specially designed teats
- problems with speech and being understood
- problems with hearing (glue ear, etc.)
- social difficulties, e.g. teasing

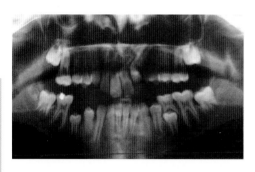

Figure 20.4 Radiograph of cleft patient. Source: Reproduced by kind permission of Jonathan Sandler.

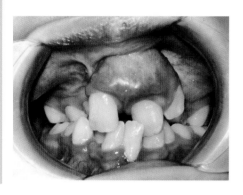

Figure 20.5 Cleft patient prior to orthodontic treatment. Source: Reproduced by kind permission of Alan Hall.

- surgical procedures, bone harvesting, osteotomies, etc.
- problems with plaque control, which affects oral hygiene
- hypoplastic, peg-shaped or absent teeth
- impacted teeth
- teeth which may have short or abnormal clinical crowns
- issues surrounding low self-esteem.

There is a considerable orthodontic interface with cleft patients to help achieve an aesthetic result which will add to the patient's self-esteem.

- at 9–10 years, they may be treated with orthodontics and bone grafting.
- at 15–18 years, they can be treated with orthodontics and an osteotomy.

To comply with national audit requirements in the UK, baseline records are taken for these patients at prescribed intervals.

Problems for the orthodontist include:

- lack of alveolar bone at site of cleft means bone grafting is needed
- teeth missing at site of cleft requires decisions on how to fill the space:
  - space closed orthodontically
  - implants
  - acid etch-retained bridges
- facial growth disrupted due to surgical interventions, e.g. maxillary retrusion
- teeth not in alignment, with upper arch narrow and deformed and tending to cross-bites and impacted teeth.

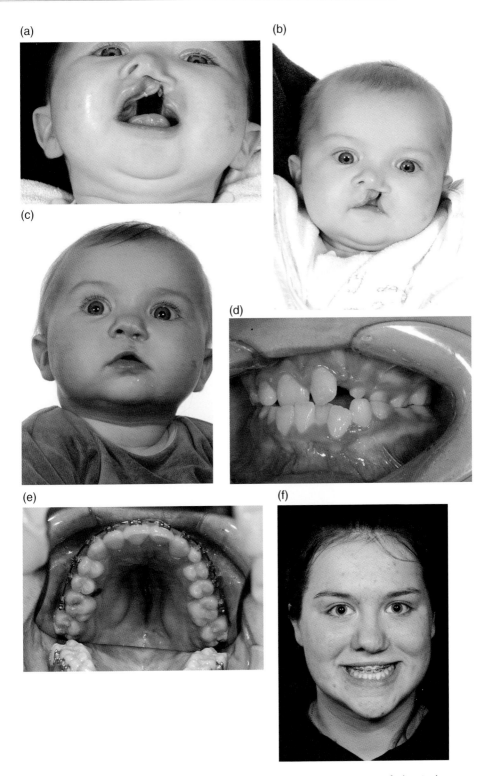

(a)

(b)

(c)

(d)

(e)

(f)

Figure 20.6 (a–f) A cleft patient's journey. Source: Reproduced by kind permission of Alex Cash.

MULTI-DISCIPLINARY ORTHODONTICS

(a)   (b)

(c)   (d)

(e)

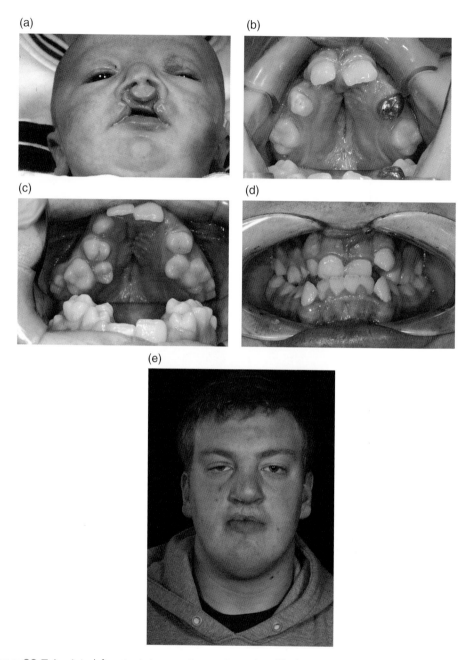

Figure 20.7 (a–e) A cleft patient's journey. Source: Reproduced by kind permission of Alex Cash.

As Figures 20.8 and 20.9 show, treatment is an amalgam of surgical intervention, dental and facial development and orthodontic skill. This is a very rewarding group of patients, whose orthodontic treatment really does make a difference to them in many ways, not least their confidence.

(a)

(d)

(e)

(b)

(c)

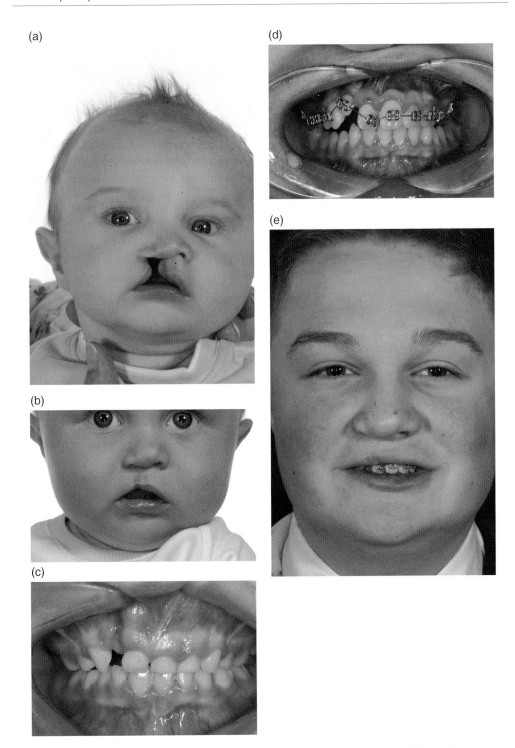

Figure 20.8 (a–e) A cleft patient's journey. Source: Reproduced by kind permission of Alex Cash.

MULTI-DISCIPLINARY ORTHODONTICS

(a)

(b)

(c)

(d)

(e)

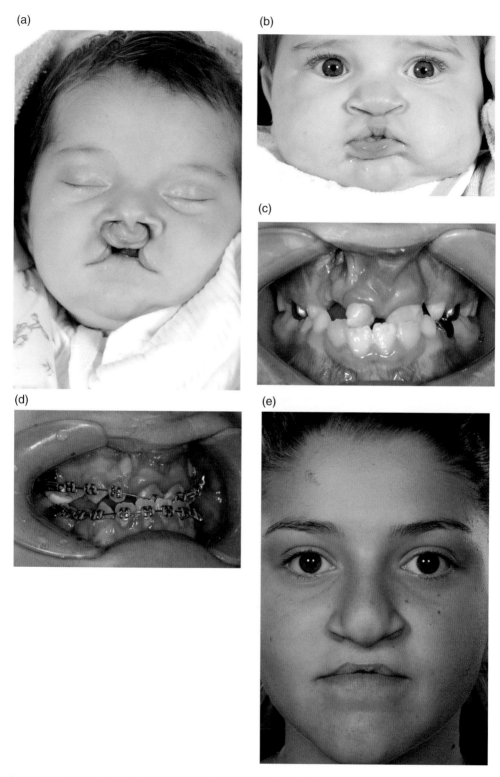

Figure 20.9 (a–e) A cleft patient's journey. Source: Reproduced by kind permission of Alex Cash.

The nurse needs to prepare the same tray layouts for these patients for every stage of appliance treatment as would be needed for patients without a cleft.

Cleft patients may need to have additional visits to other specialties as part of their treatment, e.g. speech therapy and problems with ears and noses.

In England, Wales and Northern Ireland, the Cleft Registry and Audit Network (CRANE) database was set up by the Department of Health in 2000. It holds full clinical details of adults and children with a cleft lip and/or palate. This is funded by the NHS and is held at the Royal College of Surgeons (England). Patients in Scotland come under the care of Cleft Care Scotland.

The Cleft Lip and Palate Association (CLAPA) is a representative organisation that supports all people with, or affected by, cleft lip and/or palate.

MULTI-DISCIPLINARY ORTHODONTICS

Chapter 21
Adult orthodontics

Orthodontic treatment is not confined to children and adolescents. In many ways, adults now have a greater range of treatment options open to them:

- aesthetic fixed appliances
- removable appliances
- lingual appliances
- appliance/restorative treatment, e.g. implants, bridgework
- clear aligners.

Many adult patients seek an orthodontic solution to improve their function and appearance. These patients may have discussed their concerns with their general dental practitioner (GDP). Often they may have:

- been denied access to orthodontic treatment as children
- been offered it but refused to take it up
- had orthodontics with a treatment plan that was incorrect or unsuccessful
- failed to complete treatment or to wear their retainers and the teeth relapsed.

Often, patients have been considering an orthodontic treatment option for some time before actually speaking with their dentist.

If it is a mild malocclusion involving rotations, crowding or spacing, then the patient may be referred to a specialist practitioner who has qualified as a dentist and then undertaken advanced training in order to achieve a postgraduate qualification in orthodontics.

If it is a more challenging malocclusion involving:

- an underlying skeletal asymmetry
- a complex occlusal problem
- a severe degree of crowding
- a number of congenitally missing teeth
- any untreated ectopic teeth
- signs of bone loss or a periodontal condition,

then the patient may be referred to a consultant orthodontist who has qualified as a dentist and gone on to achieve further orthodontic qualifications.

Basic Guide to Orthodontic Dental Nursing, Second Edition. Fiona Grist.
© 2020 John Wiley & Sons Ltd. Published 2020 by John Wiley & Sons Ltd.

Many adult patients now self-refer and make contact themselves. They have some advantages over younger patients because usually they:

- are compliant and keen
- know what they want
- can have interproximal enamel reduction
- have good oral hygiene
- are careful not to lose or damage their appliances.

However, they may also have some disadvantages, including:

- missing teeth
- fractured teeth which are sometimes non-vital
- root-treated teeth
- periodontal disease with resulting gum recession
- implants
- loss of alveolar ridge due to earlier extraction of teeth
- tooth surface loss
- underlying medical health problems
- finished facial growth
- teeth which have suffered trauma and have become ankylosed, i.e. fused to the surrounding tissue (these teeth cannot be moved orthodontically)
- bridgework, so in some areas, movement and space is compromised
- root resorption and low bone levels
- temporo-mandibular joint problems, e.g. pain on opening, clicking jaws
- para-functional habits, e.g. bruxism or clenching
- effects on periodontal health where the patient is a smoker
- an unhelpful wear pattern (often caused by rotations and overcrowding).

For adult patients a more socially acceptable and discreet option may include:

- fixed appliances using aesthetic brackets (these can be upper anteriors only) (Figures 21.1 and 21.2)
- removable appliances (i.e. can be removed for critical business or social meetings)
- aligners
- lingual fixed appliances (Figure 21.3).

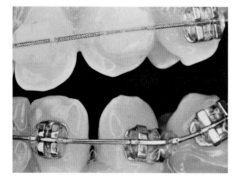

Figure 21.1 Bonding using both metal and aesthetic brackets. Source: Reproduced by kind permission of Alan Hall.

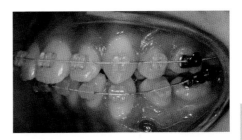

Figure 21.2 Upper and lower aesthetic brackets. Source: Reproduced by kind permission of Jonathan Sandler.

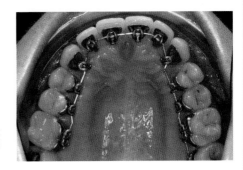

Figure 21.3 Lingual appliance with gold brackets. Source: Reproduced by kind permission of Paul Ward, British Lingual Orthodontic Society.

Patients may:

- confide that they are embarrassed to smile in public
- want to smile with more confidence
- have seen a recent photograph of themselves and realise how poor their smile is and how unhappy they are with it
- have a major life event coming, e.g. they are getting married for which they want to improve their appearance
- not have been offered the opportunity to have orthodontic treatment when they were younger
- suffer discomfort from a traumatic occlusion.

ORTHODONTIC SOLUTIONS

To rehabilitate a traumatic bite

Sometimes the patient bites in a way that is self-damaging. The longer they do it the more damage, often irreversible, is done to the teeth, gingivae and palatal soft tissue (Figure 21.4). Patients complain that they suffer more discomfort when they have a cold and the mucosa in the mouth is inflamed.

Investigating options

The patient may be investigating all the options. It can be that during the initial consultation with the dentist, the restorative options discussed included provision of crowns, bridges, veneers and implants, or a combination of these. Orthodontic treatment

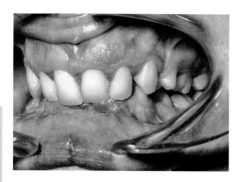

Figure 21.4 Bite stripping labial gingivae.
Source: Reproduced by kind permission of Alan Hall.

(Figure 21.5) may be proposed as an option to achieve an acceptable aesthetic solution. More and more adult patients are exploring this combination of restorative and orthodontic solutions.

Problems with eating

Adult patients who have lived for many years with crooked teeth and poor bites may complain that they feel uncomfortable eating in public. As teenagers their diet would have been less challenging and there were probably fewer social situations that highlighted these difficulties. A common complaint for some patients is that they are unable to 'bite right through a sandwich'. They manage the bread but not always a fibrous filling or lettuce. Sometimes their malocclusion does not efficiently deal with mastication and food may not have been chewed properly prior to swallowing, which may lead to perceived problems with digestion.

Oral hygiene

Some patients are very aware that their teeth are prone to trapping food after meals. For example, meat fibres or spinach leaves get caught between the teeth during and after a meal. This can be socially embarrassing. Flossing between overlapping teeth can be difficult and this may lead to localised periodontal problems. Despite a patient's best efforts, rotated and overlapping teeth tend to develop cavities and these are hard for the dentist to fill due to poor access.

Third molars

Some patients who have straight teeth worry that the eruption of wisdom teeth in their mid-twenties may cause a 'bunching' effect, known as late lower incisor crowding. There is now good evidence that late lower incisor crowding tends to happen whether or not wisdom teeth are present and is thought to be due to mandibular growth changes at the completion of facial growth. The National Institute for Health and Care Excellence (NICE) has produced guidelines which suggest that wisdom teeth should only be extracted if they are causing a proven clinical problem.

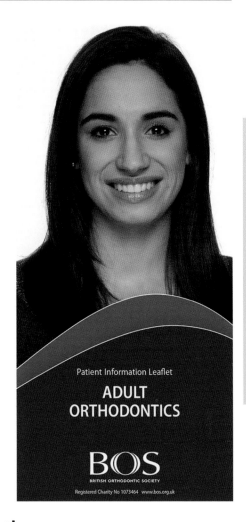

Figure 21.5 British Orthodontic Society leaflet. Source: Reproduced by kind permission of the British Orthodontic Society.

Loss of retained deciduous teeth

Some retained deciduous teeth, although severely worn down, can last into middle age. Many have no permanent tooth to act as a replacement. However, when these teeth are lost, they cause a problem: what to do with the space they have left. For some patients, the option of closing the space using braces may seem to be preferable to a bridge or an implant. Orthodontics would give them a lasting solution and there would be no need for restorative work, which may have to be replaced over time and also have an ongoing cost implication.

Alternatively, the space may need to be opened further using braces in order to place a satisfactory restoration or implant.

To assist the dentist in carrying out routine treatment

If a tilted tooth is to be used as an abutment tooth for bridgework, it may need to first be uprighted to allow good parallel preparation of the tooth. Uprighting can be achieved orthodontically. Otherwise, if it is severely tipped there is the possibility that when preparing the tooth the angle might necessitate root canal therapy.

Relapsed orthodontic treatment

Some patients have undergone orthodontic treatment as children but have relapsed for whatever reason, and problems have returned. These patients are fairly knowledgeable about what orthodontic treatment entails.

Never has the patient been supplied with such a wealth of information as on the internet. Patients come to the surgery or department with a good idea what is available and a better idea of what they want and have done their research into what is achievable and the costs. They may come in wishing for less visible appliances and have a long list of 'Can I have…?' questions.

However, for many adult patients, orthodontic treatment must have one really important feature: that preferably the appliance is not visible when worn and can be removed when necessary. It can also be left in its box for that special presentation, speech or gala event. Enter the aligner!

Aligners are popular with adults because they:

- are less visible
- can be taken out for special occasions, e.g. meetings, dates
- are easy to use and don't affect speech
- can be worn all the time (apart from when eating or drinking liquids other than water) (Figure 21.6).

Treatment with aligners is covered in Chapter 19. However, adults have different needs and aspirations from children, requiring:

- more discussion and explanation, PowerPoint presentations, and explanation of the treatment process using demonstration models
- visual presentations
- written leaflets.

With adult patients, treatment may appear similar to that for children but their treatment plans are often custom-made for them. Some adults may choose to have severely rotated teeth treated but leave a diastema. This would normally be closed in a younger patient but, as this has become part of their accepted appearance, it is not seen as requiring correction – it is part of them. Also, having had previous treatment involving extractions, options may be limited.

Adults are focused, keen and self -motivating.

- oral hygiene is rarely an issue, although staining from black coffee and red wine can be a problem.
- they can see the benefits and value of having the treatment.
- they are not going to take risks with diet, oral hygiene or not wearing the appliances as instructed.
- they are very rewarding patients to treat and they value their smile, albeit arriving a few years later than might have been the case.

Some fixed appliance therapy is available which offers very short treatment times and is often known as short-term orthodontics (STO). For example, Six Month Smiles™ certified practitioners provide treatment that focuses primarily on the anterior teeth. Using standard

ADULT ORTHODONTICS

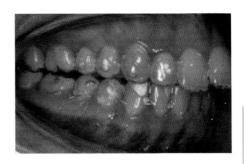

Figure 21.6 Aligners. Source: Reproduced by kind permission of Jonathan Sandler.

orthodontic mechanics, their emphasis is on the aesthetics of the teeth rather than on the position of the bite. They use small tooth-coloured brackets and NiTi wire, with short visits every 4–5 weeks for adjustment. After the appliance is removed, either a removable clear retainer or a bonded retainer is supplied.

Fastbraces™ is an alternative to removable aligners and traditional fixed appliances. Using triangular rather than square brackets and heat-activated wire, treatment time is shorter than conventional fixed appliances because there are limited treatment aims for milder cases.

The growing numbers of adults seeking an improved smile could ensure that the adult population seeking an orthodontic solution will continue to expand and develop.

ADULT ORTHODONTICS

Chapter 22

Mandibular advancement devices

Increasingly in recent years, doctors, dentists, respiratory physicians and ear, nose and throat (ENT) surgeons have been seeing patients who are worried that their husband, wife, partner, friend or relative suffers disturbed sleep and/or snore. They are concerned about:

- the noise from snoring, which can range from gentle and rhythmic to very loud
- a tendency to 'stop breathing' when asleep, called obstructive sleep apnoea (OSA). The patient stops mid snore for a few seconds, snorts or gasps and wakes themselves up, and then falls asleep again, and this can be repeated several times in an hour.

Very often it is not the patient who complains. They may feel tired but they do not always have broken sleep. It is the person who is kept awake that often encourages the snorer to seek advice.

The first step is for the snorer to see their own general practitioner (GP) to see what help is available. The GP may then refer these patients to a sleep clinic, usually at their local hospital where they are assessed by a physician and a specialist sleep nurse. In recent years there has been a rise in the number of sleep clinics as there is greater focus on the effects of sleep deprivation on both physical and mental health and well-being. To emphasise, it is not only the patient with the problem that suffers, as those around them may also experience poor-quality broken sleep.

The snorer completes an Epworth Sleepiness Test, in which patients rate how they react in certain situations by choosing the most appropriate number from the following scale:

- 0: would never doze or sleep
- 1: slight chance of dozing or sleeping
- 2: chance of dozing or sleeping
- 3: high chance of dozing or sleeping.

The situations include:

- sitting and reading
- watching TV
- sitting inactive in a public place
- travelling as a passenger in a car for more than an hour

Basic Guide to Orthodontic Dental Nursing, Second Edition. Fiona Grist.
© 2020 John Wiley & Sons Ltd. Published 2020 by John Wiley & Sons Ltd.

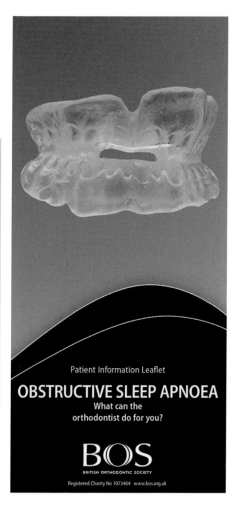

Patient Information Leaflet

OBSTRUCTIVE SLEEP APNOEA
What can the
orthodontist do for you?

BOS
BRITISH ORTHODONTIC SOCIETY
Registered Charity No 1073464   www.bos.org.uk

Figure 22.1 British Orthodontic Society leaflet. Source: Reproduced by kind permission of British Orthodontic Society.

- lying down in the afternoon
- sitting and talking to someone
- sitting after lunch (no alcohol)
- stopping for a few minutes while driving, e.g. at traffic lights.

The score from each situation is added up and the total is the patient's Epworth score. If the Epworth score is greater than 10, the patient may also suffer from OSA.

They may also be given:

- a medical examination
- a nasoendoscopy
- an overnight sleep study.

Some children and teenagers snore. This is often the result of:

- mouth breathing
- large tonsils.

By the end of the mixed dentition/early second dentition, when other facial structures relative to the tonsils have grown, the problem usually disappears.

However, for adults diagnosed with OSA and/or snoring, their problem does not go away.

SOCIAL PROBLEMS

Snoring has obvious detrimental effects, including (but not limited to):

- an adverse effect on patients' social life
- marital problems, from sleeping apart in separate rooms to sleeping on the couch and even to separation and divorce
- poor quality sleep, which affects concentration, reaction times, ability to cope, etc.
- sleep deprivation and tiredness experienced by the patient and those around them, which affects social interaction, tolerance, moods, etc.
- daytime drowsiness, often while travelling or driving
- repercussions on their job, e.g. it may jeopardise their driving licence
- loss of vitality, more time spent inactive, lack of energy, lack of enthusiasm (too tired to join in)
- social embarrassment, e.g. fellow hotel guests complaining or asking to move rooms
- problems during holidays with a partner (having to book two separate rooms)
- sleeping on aircraft, trains or other public places, etc.

Symptoms can include:

- raised blood pressure
- strain on the heart
- difficulty in concentration, sometimes affecting memory
- dry mouths, aggravating gingival/gum conditions
- depression, never feeling on top of things
- loss of libido.

These are areas which can have a major effect on people's daily lives.

WHAT CAUSES THE SNORING NOISE?

Snoring usually emanates as a noise in the back of the throat as a result of a turbulent airflow.

During sleep:

- the muscles of the face, mouth, tongue and neck relax
- the breathing passages narrow
- the tongue drops back, encroaching on the airway space
- the soft palate 'flutters' causing a noise.

MANDIBULAR ADVANCEMENT DEVICES

Factors that make the problem worse include:

- being overweight, especially in men as they carry excess weight around their necks
- drinking alcohol, especially last thing at night
- going to sleep after a heavy meal
- taking muscle relaxants (e.g. sleeping medication)
- anatomical features such as retrognathia (receding lower jaw).

WHAT ARE THE SOLUTIONS?

- try to reduce excess weight
- reduce intake of alcohol
- take more exercise.

Self-prescribing and over-the-counter remedies

There are a variety of remedies sold 'off the shelf' which are not worn in the mouth. These include (but are not limited to):

- nasal strips worn over the nose
- nasal sprays
- nasal drops
- nasal expanders
- herbal pillows
- humidifiers
- ready-made mandibular advancement devices.

The commercial devices are sold to wear in the mouth but because they are not made to fit the individual patient but are 'one size fits all', they have limited results. These appliances have the advantage of being:

- easily available
- inexpensive.

The appliances also have disadvantages, such as:

- poor fitting
- limited length of use
- bulky
- affect the occlusion
- patients don't persevere wearing them.

Some patients even try hypnotherapy to see if this can help.

Continuous positive airway pressure masks

These are prescribed mainly for OSA patients from the specialist sleep clinic.

MANDIBULAR ADVANCEMENT DEVICES

A continuous positive airway pressure (CPAP) mask can be tried. This consists of a mask that fits over the nose and air is supplied under pressure from a pump. Although considered the gold standard treatment, it does have some disadvantages.

Some patients:

- find these bulky
- report feeling a little claustrophobic while wearing the mask
- wake up with a dry mouth
- dislike the pressure on their faces
- report that the sound of the pump used to circulate the air is noisy and keeps them, and possibly their partner, awake
- consider them non-portable, making them difficult to take on holiday because they are bulky in luggage and not always easy to use in hotels.

One has only to look online to see the huge variety of devices on offer for patients to buy. Many orthodontic companies now market their own. When asked, many patients will tell of a long search trying many devices in search of a solution.

Custom-made mandibular advancement devices for the patient

The patient can have a device made specifically for them. The purpose of the device is to position the lower jaw forward. As the tongue is attached to the floor of the mouth, this is also automatically brought forward. By doing this, the airway at the back of the throat widens and the tongue does not tend to block it, so air can pass more easily. The flow of air when the patient is sleeping is improved and the noise reduces or disappears.

A number of appliances are available, ranging from the complex and expensive to the relatively basic and inexpensive to produce. They all work using the same principle.

These are variously known as:

- mandibular advancement devices
- mandibular advancement splints
- mandibular repositioning splints
- functional appliances (twin block) which postures the lower jaw forwards
- thermo-formed splints.

At the top of the range, these appliances have baseplates made from:

- chrome cobalt (a very strong light alloy metal)
- gold.

These appliances:

- are smaller
- are more closely fitting
- provide more room for the tongue.

At the other end of the scale, the simplest of these devices is the thermo-formed splint.

These appliances:

- look like a sportsman's mouthguard
- fit on the upper and lower teeth and position the lower jaw forwards

- are easy to wear
- have a central anterior opening to allow patients to breathe through their mouths, if necessary
- are made of ethylene vinyl acetate (EVA)
- can be made relatively quickly in the laboratory
- are relatively inexpensive because of the costs of the materials used.

In addition to referrals from doctors, dentists and specialist sleep study centres, orthodontists in hospitals also receive referrals from their colleagues such as respiratory consultants and ENT consultants, who:

- have medically assessed these OSA and snorer patients and wish them to have such a device
- have found their patient unable to tolerate a CPAP machine and are trying an alternative.

In the dental surgery at the assessment appointment, care is taken to record the amount of mandibular protrusion the patient can comfortably tolerate and to check that the patient has free movement of the temporo-mandibular joints (TMJs). They must also have an adequate number of teeth.

When making and following up a thermo-formed mandibular advancement device, three visits are needed and the patient is then referred back to their dentist or doctor with a report.

WHAT IS NEEDED

At the first appointment, the nurse needs to prepare:

- *the patient's clinical notes*
- *upper and lower impression trays*
- *beading or ribbon wax to extend them if necessary*
- *alginate, bowl and spatula*
- *wax for squash bite and postured bite*
- *method of softening wax (blow torch, flame or hot water)*
- *container of cold water for cooling the postured bite*
- *bowl in case of gagging reflex*
- *mouthwash and tissues*
- *impression disinfectant solution*
- *sealed plastic bag for transit*
- *laboratory instruction sheet.*

NB The device (Figures 22.2 and 22.3) is intended to hold the lower jaw forward, thereby preventing the tongue from falling back and obstructing the flow of air to the sleeping patient. Accordingly, the second bite recording is taken with the lower jaw in this protruded position. Care will be taken when designing the appliance to leave a space between the upper and lower parts so that mouth breathers will be able to inhale.

MANDIBULAR ADVANCEMENT DEVICES

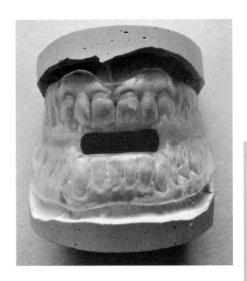

Figure 22.2 Mandibular advancement device. Source: Reproduced by kind permission of Alan Hall.

THE PROCEDURE

The nurse needs to assist the clinician to:

- *ensure that the patient and staff are wearing personal protective equipment*
- *seat the patient comfortably in the chair, sitting upright for preference*
- *prepare wax bites, one single thickness, and the other two to four thicknesses, depending on the occlusion*
- *provide a bowl of cold water (after the postured bite is taken, it must be taken out, cooled and re-inserted to check it is correct)*
- *make sure that the trays are well extended, using beading or ribbon wax*
- *mix upper and lower alginate impressions*
- *immerse the impressions and wax bites in disinfectant solution as per manufacturer's instructions*
- *fill in laboratory instruction sheet*
- *send both to the technician.*

When the technician has made the appliance, the patient returns for the second appointment to fit the device.

At the second appointment, the nurse needs to prepare:

- *the patient's notes, with the Medical Devices certificate completed*
- *the patient's model box*
- *the device*
- *a mouth mirror and ruler on a tray*
- *a suitable container for the patient to take home and use for storing the device when it is not in the mouth*
- *a hand mirror to show the patient the best method to insert and remove the device*
- *a patient instruction leaflet, giving instructions on cleaning, storage, etc.*

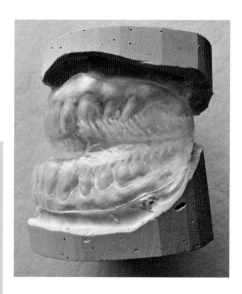

Figure 22.3 Lateral view of mandibular advancement device. Source: Reproduced by kind permission of Alan Hall.

Then:

- *ensure that the patient and staff are wearing personal protective equipment*
- *seat the patient comfortably in the chair*
- *once the device has been fitted, make sure that the patient:*
  - *can take it in and out themselves*
  - *knows how to clean it*
  - *is given written instructions*
  - *is supplied with a rigid box for storing it when not in use.*

Like aligners, it is recommended to clean the device using cold water and a little liquid soap. Toothpaste and brushes are abrasive and harm the surface.

On the third appointment the nurse needs to prepare only:

- *the patient's clinical notes*
- *the patient's model box*
- *mouth mirror.*

The patient does not need to sit in the dental chair for this as this appointment is to:

- give feedback
- assess any difficulties
- quantify how successful it has been.

If there has been adequate improvement, the patient continues to wear the device. If there has not and the patient is not able or prepared to wear it, the treatment is discontinued. A letter is written to inform the referring doctor and their dentist that this is the case.

Further consideration regarding alternative options available to the patient will then have to be discussed.

OUTCOME

Advantages

- the success rate for these appliances is very good.
- they are disinfected in a simple solution of Milton antiseptic.
- they do not require a power supply to make them work.
- as it is a non-invasive procedure, it is reversible.
- when successful it will have made a great improvement in the quality of life for OSA sufferers, snorers and their families.

Disadvantages

- they do not last indefinitely.
- they can become stained.
- the join between the upper and lower components has a tendency to split.

There are an increasing number of clinics and practices that deal exclusively with problems associated with poor-quality sleep, their causes, symptoms and remedies. They offer a wide range of treatment options and are available to patients to access themselves. Their details can be found by looking on the internet.

CONCLUSION

Mandibular advancement devices can:

- reduce noise
- help to provide quality sleep
- help reduce levels of tiredness
- benefit general health
- help the patient's self-esteem
- benefit relationships with partners.

They are non-invasive and if successful produce a good outcome, providing immediate relief for patients, their partners and those around them. If unsuccessful, the patient has not been permanently affected by an irreversible process; however, this cohort of patients has a real social and health-related problem.

MANDIBULAR ADVANCEMENT DEVICES

Chapter 23

Study models and digital storage of records

At the beginning of every orthodontic patient's treatment, baseline records are taken to aid assessment and monitor progress and for medico-legal purposes. These include:

- study models
- radiographs
- intra-oral and extra-oral photographs.

These must all be carefully stored as they contain confidential data that must be protected.

Study models are a very important part of the patient's treatment and need to be available to the clinician at every appointment. There are two methods of producing them: traditional and digital.

The traditional method involves taking:

- upper and lower alginate or rubber-based impressions
- a wax squash bite to record the occlusion.

The technicians cast these in the laboratory, using either a plaster or stone mix. Orthodontic models are trimmed in a specific way (Figure 23.1).

During a course of treatment, numerous sets of impressions can be taken, including study, stage, working, coordination and planning models, and wafer, debonding and final impressions.

STUDY MODELS

These are kept in the patient's model box, and used for reference and as a record of the patient's occlusion at that time.

STAGE MODELS

These are taken at the end of a stage of treatment, e.g. when a patient has completed the expansion stage or functional stage of treatment and is going into fixed appliances.

Basic Guide to Orthodontic Dental Nursing, Second Edition. Fiona Grist.
© 2020 John Wiley & Sons Ltd. Published 2020 by John Wiley & Sons Ltd.

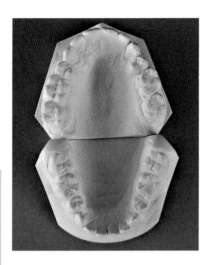

Figure 23.1 Example of the method of trimming orthodontic models. Source: Reproduced by kind permission of Alan Hall.

WORKING MODELS

The working model is the model on which the technician makes the appliance.

CO-ORDINATION MODELS

When the pre-surgical orthodontic phase of treatment is completed, impressions are taken to confirm that the teeth have been moved into the planned position and that the upper and lower arches will be co-ordinated in the planned post-operative position.

PLANNING MODELS

When the patient is to have orthognathic surgery, models are mounted on articulators. The models are cut and remounted to the planned occlusion to enable the surgeon to see the movement required at the operation. Also, to aid planning and assessment (e.g. for cases of hypodontia and some complex orthodontic cases), a Kesling set-up is fabricated to prescription in the laboratory. This is a procedure whereby individual teeth are cut off a working model and reset to the prescribed position to simulate future orthodontic tooth movements.

WAFER IMPRESSIONS

The models from these impressions are used to make the acrylic wafer that is used by the maxillofacial surgeon in theatre during an osteotomy.

DEBONDING IMPRESSIONS

These are taken when the appliances are removed. The technician will cast two sets of models: one set is used as working models for making retainers and another as study models.

FINAL IMPRESSIONS

These are taken at the end of treatment, when the patient is discharged.

Many of these models must be kept as permanent records. The initial and final models are a medico-legal record of:

- pre-treatment
- post-treatment.

At the end of treatment, these models can be scored to measure the percentage change that treatment has achieved. This is done using an occlusal index called Peer Assessment Rating (PAR), which is discussed in detail in Chapter 3.

When monitoring the percentage improvement that has been achieved by orthodontic intervention, five areas are considered:

- anterior segments, upper and lower
- buccal occlusion, right and left
- overbite or open bite
- overjet
- centre line.

Because the models for each patient need to be available at each visit, they must be stored in an easily accessible system. There are many excellent systems; what works well for an individual surgery or unit is the best for them and the one they should choose.

The system adopted is often governed by:

- the number of patients under treatment, i.e. the number of boxes needed
- the size and accessibility of the storage area.

The patient's individual box number can be stored:

- on their computer notes
- on their paper notes
- on a computer spreadsheet
- in an 'index of model boxes' book, kept in the model store room.

One suggested method is to:

- file boxes in numerical order and cross-reference in alphabetical order
- use an easily accessible racking or shelving system to maximise space and save time
- write the number of each patient's box in their notes
- record on computer in the patient's details.

STUDY MODELS AND
DIGITAL STORAGE OF RECORDS

Given that there can be many hundreds of boxes in current use at any one time, a separate cross-reference book or spreadsheet is kept with details entered both ways:

- patient names listed alphabetically at the front of the book
- patient numbers listed numerically at the back of the book.

If one entry is overlooked, the other usually locates the models. It is a belt and braces method that works. If a patient's models are misfiled or incorrectly recorded, it takes a lot of time to find them!

All the patient's details, i.e. name and reference number (if applicable), age and clinician, are noted:

- on a changeable label on the front of the box or
- on the inside of the lid of the box,

In order to comply with patient confidentiality and data protection regulations currently in force, the names of patients must not be visible to other patients either in the surgery or in storage.

All the patient's models should be boxed (Figure 23.2), before and after treatment and at other times if there has been more than one phase of treatment, e.g. a functional appliance before a fixed.

At the completion of treatment, when the patient is no longer under supervised retention, the patient's models are transferred from 'current' storage to the archive file. This can then:

- free up that number for another patient and the numbers will still run sequentially
- prevent that number becoming 'dead' and new patients having ever higher numbers.

Because of the number of boxes stored in the out-of-treatment archive:

- they must be filed in alphabetical order, and
- in the year that treatment was completed and the patient was discharged.

This makes it easier to identify and dispose of models when they are no longer needed.

When the decision has been made to destroy models, this must be done carefully. They must have all trace of the patient's personal details removed and must not be put in clinical or commercial waste. This is because they contain gypsum, which must not go to landfill sites alongside biodegradable waste due to the production of hydrogen sulphide gas. Local authorities will have guidelines on preferred procedures. As is the case with all records, the

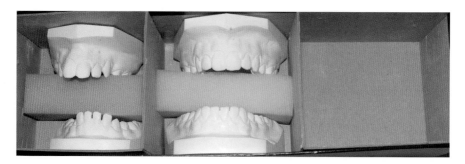

Figure 23.2 Models stored in box. Source: Reproduced by kind permission of Alan Hall.

destruction of models must be noted in the log book and patient records; this proves that they no longer exist rather than have been lost or mislaid.

Orthodontic models are part of the patient's records and must be kept according to current guidelines. Noting the patient's date of birth on the box can be helpful when calculating when the models should be discarded. The patient's notes must record the date models have been:

- moved from one storage site to another
- discarded.

Patients who have had long or multidisciplinary treatments often have more than one box. Some boxes have the upper and lower model stored apart (Figure 23.3); some have them stored together, with a foam pad between the teeth so that the occlusal surfaces are not damaged.

When choosing the site of your archive storage area, remember that the contents of several hundred boxes weigh a ton!

Boxes for cleft patients or patients who underwent orthognathic surgery can be marked with an additional coloured label for ease of identification and retrieval. Boxes for cleft lip and palate patients should also be specially marked because their models must be kept for a longer period and records are taken at particular ages and intervals for national audit purposes. Patients who have undergone surgery may also have a maxillofacial storage box as well.

However, technology marches on and the days of this traditional method may well be numbered. Enter the digital study model!

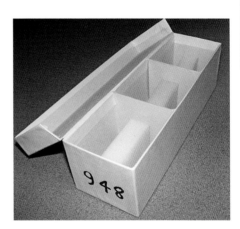

Figure 23.3 Model box. Source: Reproduced by kind permission of Alan Hall.

THE DIGITAL METHOD

Collection and management of three-dimensional rendered orthodontic study models

One of the fastest-growing areas in the provision of orthodontics is that of digital technology and its various innovations and uses. It changes so rapidly and in so many directions that its applications are far- reaching. One of these areas is the creation and storage of orthodontic records.

Study models are an intrinsic part of the management of orthodontic treatment, for planning, monitoring and evaluating. Digital study models can be obtained either:

- using equipment to intra-orally scan the patient and record the occlusion
- by extra-orally scanning existing conventional impressions or cast models.

There are some obvious advantages to the digital method, including the following.

- there are significant savings in surgery and staff time and of impression materials, wax and decontamination sundries.
- there are savings in laboratory time and materials and thus of laboratory costs.
- study models are no longer at risk of being damaged.
- study models are no longer at risk of being mislaid or misfiled.
- patients prefer this method, especially the ones who gag.

There is one very obvious reason why this method does not have widespread use yet: the initial start-up costs. However, in time, what is now only for the few will become mainstream for all.

Like graph pencils (once vital for making a cephalometric tracing, but now largely overtaken by bespoke software programs) the time may come when trays are no longer required for taking an impression.

The new technology has benefits but needs new systems. The next step is developing and organising secure sites and protocols for the collection and safe storage of all data to comply with both the current legislation and data protection legislation. As technology moves at a rapid rate, you need to keep abreast of developments.

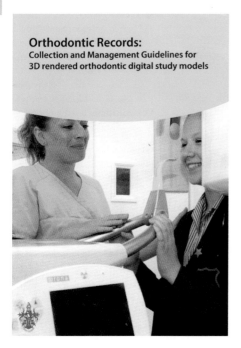

Orthodontic Records:
Collection and Management Guidelines for
3D rendered orthodontic digital study models

Figure 23.4 British Orthodontic Society guidelines for digital study models. Source: Reproduced by kind permission of the British Orthodontic Society.

STUDY MODELS AND
DIGITAL STORAGE OF RECORDS

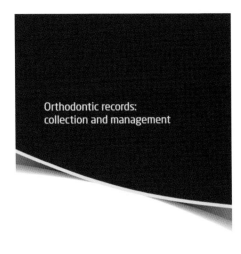

Figure 23.5 British Orthodontic Society guideline for orthodontic records. Source: Reproduced by kind permission of the British Orthodontic Society.

The British Orthodontic Society (BOS) publishes the excellent *Orthodontic Records: Collection and Management Guidelines of 3D rendered orthodontic digital study models*. It covers three areas:

- the quality of the scan
- intercuspal accuracy
- security of the data over the course of treatment and possible long-term retention (Figure 23.4).

This was updated by the Clinical Governance Directorate of the British Orthodontic Society in 2017. Recommendations may change in the light of new evidence. This BOS guideline will provide up-to-date comprehensive in-depth information on all these areas.

As the digital format for taking and storing the other two main types of clinical records (i.e. clinical photography and radiography) becomes the norm, it will be also be a rapidly changing area. Everything written today will be out of date in a matter of years, maybe even months.

The BOS guideline *Orthodontic Records: Collection and Management* covers all aspects of taking, securely storing and disposal of this data, plus the protocols and legal requirements that must be observed (Figure 23.5). This was updated by the Clinical Governance Directorate of the British Orthodontic Society in 2015. Recommendations may change in the light of new evidence.

Chapter 24

Descriptions and photographs of the most commonly used instruments and auxiliaries

Acid etch	Chemical gel used before primer to prepare tooth surface before bonding an attachment (Figure 24.1)

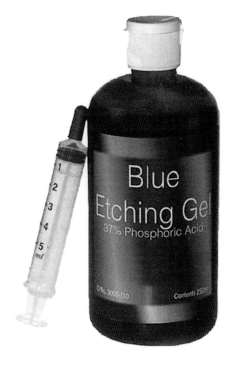

Figure 24.1

| Adams clasp (crib) | Clasp (often called a crib) used on removable appliances for retention (Figure 24.2) |

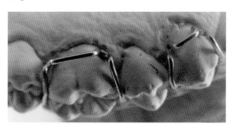

Figure 24.2

| Adams pliers | Pliers used to adjust wire components on removable appliance (Figure 24.3) |

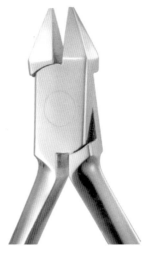

Figure 24.3

| Adhesive | Material that bonds brackets, tubes, etc. to teeth (Figure 24.4) |

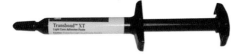

Figure 24.4
Source: Reproduced by kind permission of 3M Unitek © 2019. All rights reserved.

| Adhesive-removing pliers | Pliers with a blade that removes adhesive from tooth after debonding (Figure 24.5) |

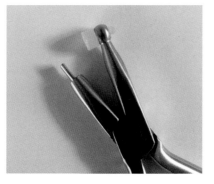

Figure 24.5

Aesthetic bracket   Less visible, non-metal bracket (Figure 24.6)

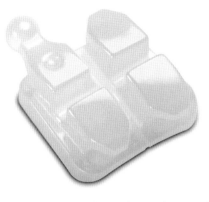

Figure 24.6

Appliance box   Box to store removable appliance when out of the mouth, e.g. sport (Figure 24.7)

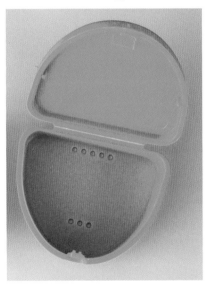

Figure 24.7

Archwire   Formed wire used in fixed appliances (Figure 24.8)

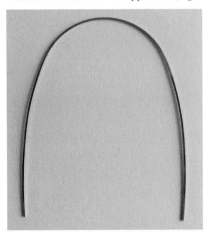

Figure 24.8

DESCRIPTIONS AND PHOTOGRAPHS OF THE MOST COMMONLY

Archwire stands   Convenient holder for many different sizes of archwire (Figure 24.9)

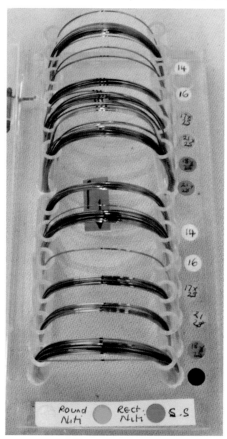

Figure 24.9

Australian wire   Type of spooled steel wire (Figure 24.10)

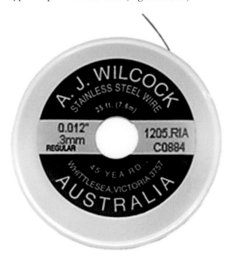

Figure 24.10

Band slitters For cutting bands to release them from tooth (Figure 24.11)

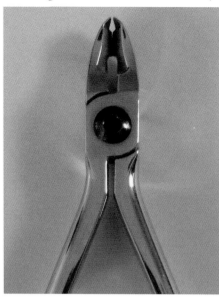

Figure 24.11

Bird-beak pliers Multi-use for removable appliances, popular, strong, has a round and a square beak (Figure 24.12)

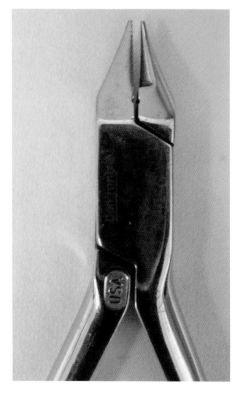

Figure 24.12

Bite stick

Nylon. Patient bites on this to fully seat metal band with triangular bite pad, which may be soft metal. Autoclavable (Figure 24.13)

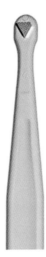

Figure 24.13

Bonded retainer

Wire or metal bar cemented to the lingual/palatal side of teeth as a fixed retainer (Figure 24.14)

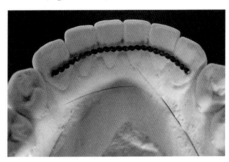

Figure 24.14

Bracket

A metal or ceramic attachment bonded to the teeth in fixed appliances through which the archwire is slotted (Figure 24.15)

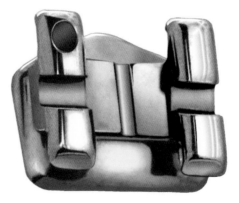

Figure 24.15

Bracket-holding tweezers   For use with direct bonding. Holds individual bracket, when placing onto tooth. Press handles together to open beak to release bracket (Figure 24.16)

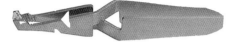

Figure 24.16

Bracket-removing pliers   For use on steel, plastic and ceramic brackets (Figure 24.17)

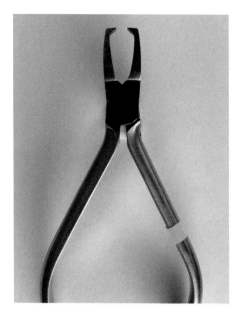

Figure 24.17

Braided wire   Wire made up of several strands braided together (Figure 24.18)

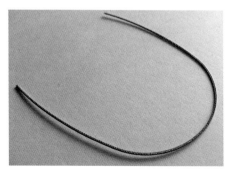

Figure 24.18

Buccal tube   Tube which can be bonded to the cheek surface of tooth or may be welded to a
                                   band. Tube can be of round or rectangular section into which the archwire fits
                                   (Figure 24.19)

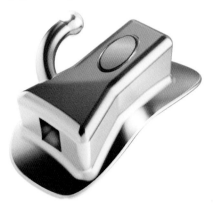

Figure 24.19

Bump-R-Sleeve   Clear sleeving, fits over archwire to prevent wire cutting into soft tissues
                                   (Figure 24.20)

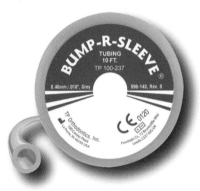

Figure 24.20
Source: Courtesy of TP
Orthodontics Bump-R-Sleeve.
Registered trademark of TP
Orthodontics Inc. All rights
reserved.

Cement   Lining material inside the band when fitted on a tooth, eliminates space
                                   between band and enamel (Figure 24.21)

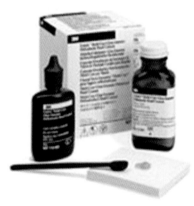

Figure 24.21
Source: By kind permission of
3M Unitek Copyright 2019.
All rights reserved.

Chain   Line of joined elastic links, available in various sizes, can be clear or coloured
                         (Figure 24.22)

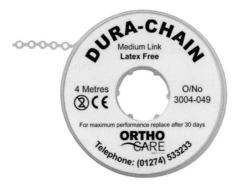

Figure 24.22

Cheek retractor   Plastic frame, keeps lips and cheeks away from teeth and gives better vision,
                         access and moisture control (Figure 24.23)

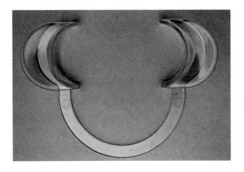

Figure 24.23

Coil (open and closed)   Sold on spools, to either open or maintain a space (Figure 24.24)

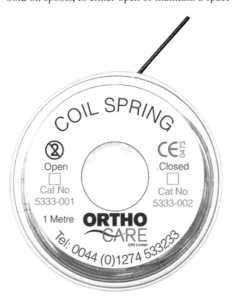

Figure 24.24

Coil spring

Fits over archwire to provide constant, gentle force when activated to open spaces between teeth or maintain spaces when passive (Figure 24.25)

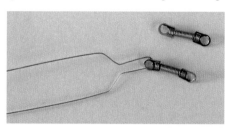

Figure 24.25

Coon's ligature-tying pliers

Pliers for tying metal ligatures, similar function to Mathieu pliers (Figure 24.26)

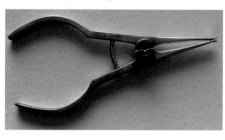

Figure 24.26

Curing light

Used to cure light-activated adhesive and cement (Figure 24.27)

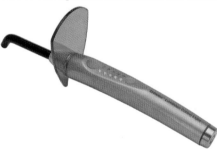

Figure 24.27
Source: By kind permission of 3M Unitek Copyright 2019. All rights reserved.

Dappen's pot

Container (disposable) for use with etch primer and prophy paste (Figure 24.28)

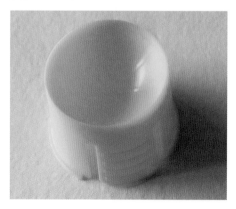

Figure 24.28

Debonding bur

Bur for removing composite from enamel (Figure 24.29)

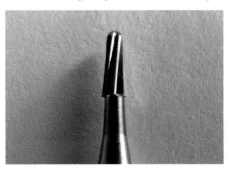

Figure 24.29

Director

Double-ended hand instrument with notches to help hold wire when ligating (Figure 24.30)

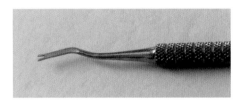

Figure 24.30

Distal end cutters

Cuts archwire flush or close to the distal end of the buccal tube. Holds the excess after cutting (Figure 24.31)

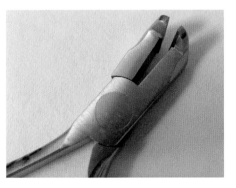

Figure 24.31

Dividers

Adjustable instrument for measuring distances between teeth (Figure 24.32)

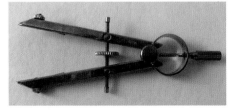

Figure 24.32

DESCRIPTIONS AND PHOTOGRAPHS
OF THE MOST COMMONLY

Elastic placer   For ease in attaching elastics (Figure 24.33)

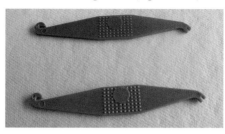

Figure 24.33

Elastomerics   Rings to secure wires onto brackets, often known as O-rings (Figure 24.34)

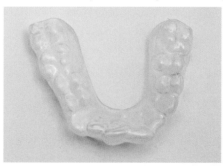

Figure 24.34

Essix retainer   Removable retainer, fits over teeth, no metal components (Figure 24.35)

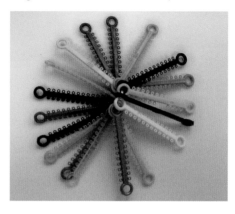

Figure 24.35

Eyelet   Bondable or weldable metal attachment, used for attaching traction (Figure 24.36)

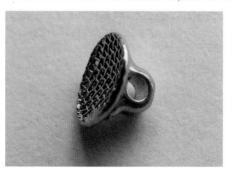

Figure 24.36

Fixed lingual retainer wire   Wire especially for fixed retainers (Figure 24.37)

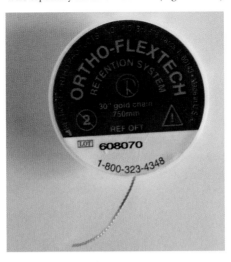

Figure 24.37

Force module separator   Another name for separating pliers (Figure 24.38)

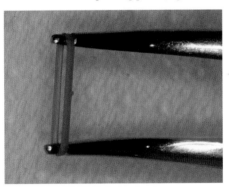

Figure 24.38

Hawley retainer   Removable retainer, acrylic baseplate with metal bow, cribs and clasps (Figure 24.39)

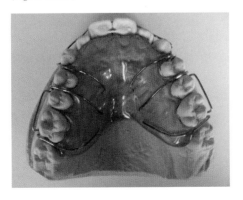

Figure 24.39

High pull head caps   Ready-made caps, to combine with headgear modules (Figure 24.40)

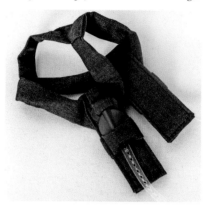

Figure 24.40

Intermaxilliary elastics   Elastics that are fitted between upper and lower dental arches (Figure 24.41)

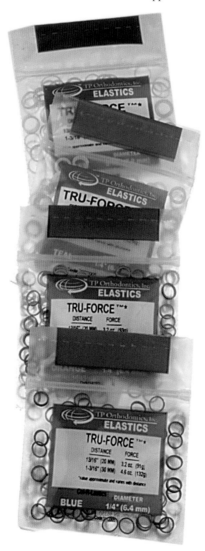

Figure 24.41
Source: Courtesy of TP
Orthodontics Tru-Force.
Registered trademark of TP
Orthodontics. All rights
reserved.

Interproximal stripper kit

For reducing contact points between the teeth (Figure 24.42)

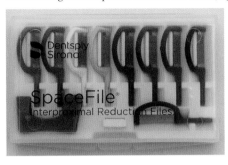

Figure 24.42

Interspace brush

Single tufted brush for cleaning around archwire (Figure 24.43)

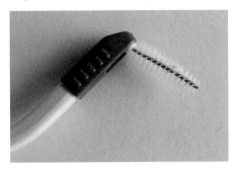

Figure 24.43

Kobayashi hook ligature

Hook-shaped end of ligature, used with intermaxillary elastics (Figure 24.44)

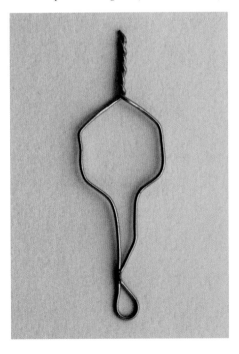

Figure 24.44

Ligature director

Double-ended hand instrument, notched, holds wire in bracket slot when ligating (Figure 24.45)

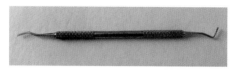

Figure 24.45

Light wire pliers

Tapered beaks, one round, one square for bending fixed appliance archwires (Figure 24.46)

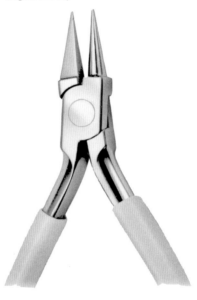

Figure 24.46

Lip bumper

Strips of rubber which fit over anterior brackets, useful for patients who play musical instruments by mouth (Figure 24.47)

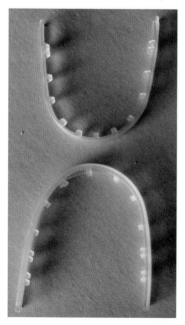

Figure 24.47

Lip retractor Same function as cheek retractors (Figure 24.48)

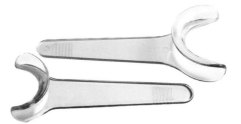

Figure 24.48

Mandibular advancement device Appliance that postures the lower jaw forward to open the airway to reduce snoring noise (Figure 24.49)

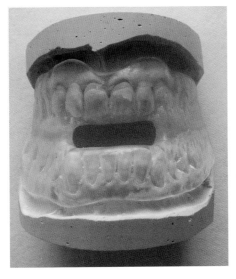

Figure 24.49

Mathieu haemostat Used to ligate wires and hold elastomerics. Ratchet lock on closing, spring-loaded, easy to turn in hand, firm grip (Figure 24.50)

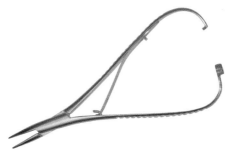

Figure 24.50

Mauns cutters

Heavy-duty pliers, used to cut wire outside the mouth, e.g. facebows (Figure 24.51)

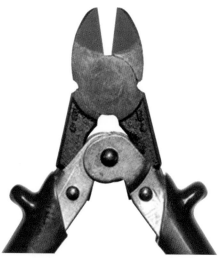

Figure 24.51

Mershon pusher

Used to seat and contour bands to teeth. Can have chunky, standard or round handle (Figure 24.52)

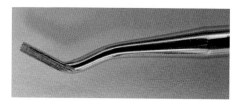

Figure 24.52

Microbrush

Disposable applicators (Figure 24.53)

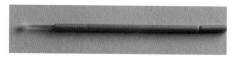

Figure 24.53

Mitchell trimmer

Double-ended multipurpose hand instrument (Figure 24.54)

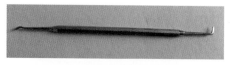

Figure 24.54

Model box

For storage of models for individual cases (Figure 24.55)

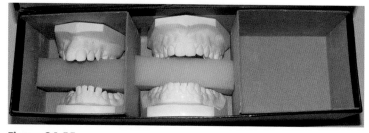

Figure 24.55

Mosquito forceps

Positive locking, to place elastomerics, ligatures, etc. Beaks smooth or serrated (Figure 24.56)

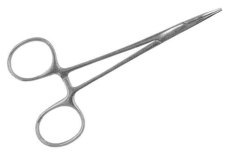

Figure 24.56

Occlusal registration bite recorders

To hold wax when recording a bite (Figure 24.57)

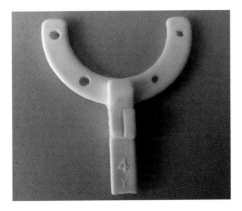

Figure 24.57

O-rings

Name given to elastomerics (Figure 24.58)

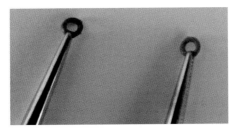

Figure 24.58

PAR ruler   Ruler used to measure occlusal indices (Figure 24.59)

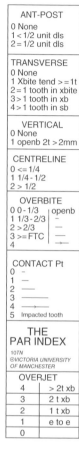

Figure 24.59
Source: By kind permission of Ortho-Care (UK) Limited and
University of Manchester.

Photographic mirrors   Double-sided, chromium-coated glass, several shapes (Figure 24.60)

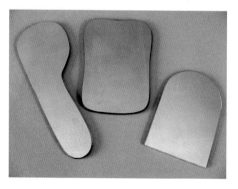

Figure 24.60

Pin and ligature cutting pliers

Cuts pins (Begg), ligatures and light wires (Figure 24.61)

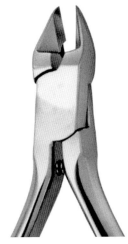

Figure 24.61

Posted archwire

Archwire that has posts attached to it, which point gingivally, used for traction (Figure 24.62)

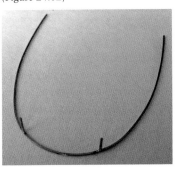

Figure 24.62

Posterior band-removing pliers

Has pad rests on occlusal surface to ease the the band off the tooth, replacement heads available (Figure 24.63)

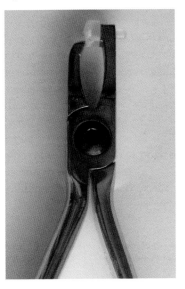

Figure 24.63

Primer

Solution applied to teeth after etchant before adhesive during bonding procedures (Figure 24.64)

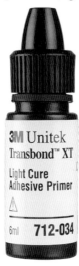

Figure 24.64
Source: Reproduced by kind permission of 3M Unitek © 2019. All rights reserved.

Retainer Brite

Kills germs, helps control calculus, keeps removable appliances clean and fresh (Figure 24.65)

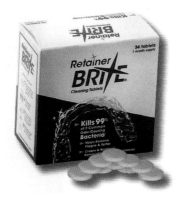

Figure 24.65
Source: By kind permission of Ortho-Care Limited (UK).

Retainer case

For storing retainers when not in mouth (Figure 24.66)

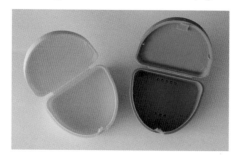

Figure 24.66

Reverse curve wire   Pre-formed archwire used to help reduce deep overbite (Figure 24.67)

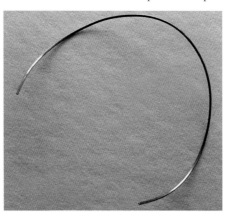

Figure 24.67

Rotation wedge   Auxiliary in fixed appliance therapy (Figure 24.68)

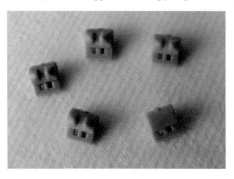

Figure 24.68

Ruler   Chrome or stainless steel, 6 inch (150 mm) (Figure 24.69)

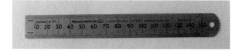

Figure 24.69

Safety facebows   For use with headgear (Figure 24.70)

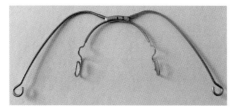

Figure 24.70

Safety glasses   Orange, for use with curing light (Figure 24.71); tinted, for general use
                              (Figure 24.72)

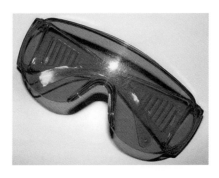

Figure 24.71

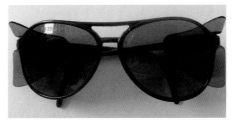

Figure 24.72

Safety swivel key   Key for turning expansion screws (Figure 24.73)

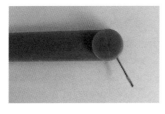

Figure 24.73

Self-etch primer   Single-use application of self-etch primer, used when bonding attachments to
                              teeth (Figure 24.74)

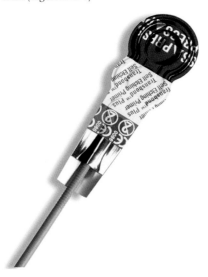

Figure 24.74
Source: By kind permission of
3M Unitek Copyright 2019. All
rights reserved.

Separating pliers

For placing separators and elastics (Figure 24.75)

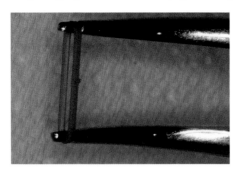

Figure 24.75

Silicone (medical grade)

To protect soft tissues from irritation by fixed appliance (Figure 24.76)

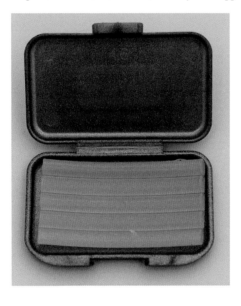

Figure 24.76

Tweed rectangular arch-forming pliers

Wire-bending pliers, for use on square and rectangular wire, use two together (Figure 24.77)

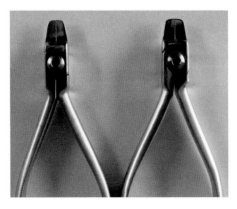

Figure 24.77

DESCRIPTIONS AND PHOTOGRAPHS
OF THE MOST COMMONLY

Twirl-on   Brand name of hand instrument used for inserting elastomerics (O-rings)
                             (Figure 24.78)

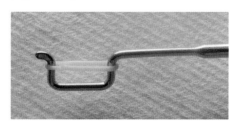

Figure 24.78

Weingart utility pliers   Serrated pads, tapering beaks, can also be angled (Figure 24.79)

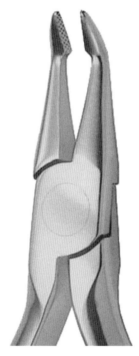

Figure 24.79

Z spring   Spring used in removable appliances (Figure 24.80)

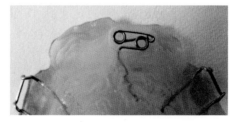

Figure 24.80

Zing String   Elastic thread used to provide traction (Figure 24.81.)

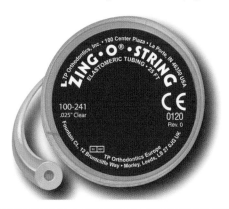

Figure 24.81
Source: Courtesy of TP
Orthodontics. Zing String is
a registered trademark of TP
Orthodontics Inc. All rights
reserved.

Chapter 25

Certificate in Orthodontic Nursing, extended duties and ongoing training

In addition to the initial National Certificate and NVQ Course and Examination, there are a variety of post-qualification courses that are available. The number of subjects covered is steadily increasing as nurses are encouraged to increase the extent of their competencies. Nurses who work in the field of orthodontics are very fortunate to have a post-qualification course in their specialty and the orthodontic profession was very supportive of its development.

WHAT IS IT?

The Certificate in Orthodontic Nursing was introduced in 2001 and is now well established as a popular postgraduate qualification. The National Examination Board for Dental Nurses (NEBDN) is its awarding body. The responsibility for registering students for this award lies with the training centres.

WHO IS ELIGIBLE TO GO ON THE COURSE?

The course is intended for dental nurses who work within orthodontics. Nurses who wish to go on to attain this certificate must:

- be registered with the General Dental Council
- be a qualified dental nurse
- have the support and written approval of their employer who will give them time off to attend the course
- validate the practical work done that is necessary to complete the Portfolio of Experience.

Basic Guide to Orthodontic Dental Nursing, Second Edition. Fiona Grist.
© 2020 John Wiley & Sons Ltd. Published 2020 by John Wiley & Sons Ltd.

THE FEE STRUCTURE FOR THE COURSE

The cost of the registration for the course and the examination fee varies between training centres. Up-to-the-minute information on this, and where the training centres are located, is available by contacting the NEBDN or by looking on the internet.

WHAT DOES THE COURSE INVOLVE?

Once on the course, nurses will need to attend lectures and instruction on the theoretical aspect of study. For this there is a comprehensive syllabus.

Delegates also need to show that they can apply this knowledge in a practical setting. For this they need to compile a Portfolio of Experience that records their competencies.

The written **Examination Paper** consists of two parts:

- paper A, made up of multiple-choice questions
- paper B, consisting of short answers to structured questions.

The exam is taken at the nurse's designated training centre and is independently assessed by NEBDN examiners.

The **Portfolio of Experience** has two parts.

Part 1: Log Sheet

Students must record their involvement in the treatment of at least 50 cases. Of these:

- 10 must be in removable appliance therapy, including five patients with functional appliances
- 10 patients in fixed appliance therapy.

Part 2: Case Studies

The student must produce two detailed case studies. These must be:

- to advise a patient on oral hygiene, and instruction on how to look after their orthodontic appliance
- to follow a patient whose orthodontic treatment was part of an interdisciplinary interface.

THE SYLLABUS FOR THE CERTIFICATE IN ORTHODONTIC NURSING

SECTION ONE   ANATOMICAL STRUCTURES RELATIVE TO ORTHODONTICS
1.1   Define the function and structure of the:
    1.1.1   muscles of mastication
    1.1.2   muscles of facial expression and soft tissues
    1.1.3   tongue
    1.1.4   maxilla and mandible
1.2   Describe the:
    1.2.1   structure and morphology of deciduous teeth and their eruption dates
    1.2.2   structure and morphology of permanent teeth and their eruption dates
    1.2.3   growth and development of the mandible and maxilla
    1.2.4   basic principles of the biology of teeth movement

SECTION TWO   CLASSIFICATION OF MALOCCLUSION
2.1   Describe and identify:
    2.1.1   skeletal classification
    2.1.2   incisor
    2.1.3   molar
    2.1.4   define diagnostic terms, e.g. overbite, crossbite

SECTION THREE   ORTHODONTIC TREATMENT
3.1   Understand the aims and limitations of orthodontic treatment
3.2   Understand the risks and benefits of orthodontic treatment
3.3   Explain how treatment progress is monitored
3.4   Discuss finishing and detailing techniques
3.5   Explain the function, need and duration of retention

SECTION FOUR   ORTHODONTIC RECORDS
4.1   Describe:
    4.1.1   the importance of orthodontic record taking
    4.1.2   the use of written assessment records and medical history
    4.1.3   effective methods of clinical photography
    4.1.4   the types of radiographs and their relevance in orthodontic treatment
    4.1.5   an effective system for the storage of orthodontic models
4.2   Demonstrate:
    4.2.1   effective methods of clinical photography
    4.2.2   completion of cephalometric tracing, digitising and measurement
    4.2.3   the chairside procedure for the production of study models

SECTION FIVE   ORTHODONTIC APPLIANCES
5.1   Active and passive removable appliances:
    5.1.1   explain the indications
    5.1.2   describe the advantages and disadvantages
    5.1.3   describe the components of an appliance
    5.1.4   describe the construction of an appliance

CERTIFICATE IN ORTHODONTIC NURSING

5.1.5   describe the different types of appliances and their uses
5.1.6   describe the chairside procedures required to produce a working model
5.1.7   identify the instruments and equipment used during the construction of appliances and describe and demonstrate their use during the procedure
5.1.8   identify the materials required during the procedure and demonstrate their use
5.1.9   explain the nature of the advice given to patients on the care of appliances
5.1.10 be able to identify the levels of damage to appliances and their potential for repair

5.2 Fixed appliances:
5.2.1   explain the indications
5.2.2   describe the advantages and disadvantages
5.2.3   describe the different types of appliances and their uses
5.2.4   describe the components of an appliance and the importance of brackets and bands
5.2.5   describe the construction of an appliance
5.2.6   describe the chairside procedures required to construct appliances
5.2.7   demonstrate the orientation of brackets
5.2.8   describe the faults which can occur when positioning brackets and their effects
5.2.9   describe and define the types and use of orthodontic wire
5.2.10 describe the use of intra-oral elastics and other auxiliaries
5.2.11 identify the instruments and equipment used during the construction of appliances and describe and demonstrate their use during the procedure
5.2.12 identify the materials used during the procedure and demonstrate their use
5.2.13 explain the nature of the advice given to patients on the care of appliances

5.3 Extra-oral traction:
5.3.1   describe the principles of use and directional force
5.3.2   identify the components of extra-oral traction
5.3.3   identify types and describe the fitting of safety headgear

SECTION SIX CROSS-INFECTION CONTROL IN ORTHODONTICS
6.1 Describe the orthodontic team's responsibility in relation to:
6.1.1   cross-infection
6.1.2   health and safety
6.1.3   sharps policy
6.1.4   COSHH

SECTION SEVEN INTERDISCIPLINARY CARE
7.1 Describe the role of orthodontics in the management of the combined orthodontic/surgical patient
7.2 The restorative/orthodontic interface
7.3 Describe the classification, aetiology and prevalence of cleft lip and palate

SECTION EIGHT LABORATORY SKILLS
8.1 Describe the laboratory stages required for appliances and the need for effective communication with the dental laboratory
8.2 Demonstrate the preparation and casting of study models

SECTION NINE ORAL HEALTH IN RELATION TO THE CARE AND MANAGEMENT OF APPLIANCES

9.1 Describe how diet may affect oral health and how the orthodontic team can help the patient to improve it

9.2 Demonstrate effective communication skills on the following:

    9.2.1 advice on the range of food and drinks which are liable to cause caries and the potential risks involved with orthodontic appliances

    9.2.2 encourage a patient to follow an efficient dental health routine whilst wearing fixed or removable appliances

    9.2.3 monitoring, evaluation and progression

SECTION TEN ORTHODONTIC STOCK CONTROL

10.1 Define and discuss effective stock control and maintenance of orthodontic materials and medicaments

10.2 Define and discuss control and maintenance of orthodontic instruments and equipment

SECTION ELEVEN MEDICO-LEGAL

11.1 Describe the importance of data protection and access to patient records in relation to their own responsibilities and those of other team members' responsibilities (e.g. General Data Protection 2018 and Access to Medical Records Act)

11.2 Describe the importance of keeping up-to-date orthodontic records and the medico-legal implications of storing orthodontic records

11.3 Describe how the practice of orthodontics is regulated and how these regulations affect the orthodontic dental nurse and other members of the orthodontic team

11.4 Explain what is meant by the term 'informed consent'

SECTION TWELVE ORTHODONTIC INDICES AND CLINICAL GOVERNANCE

12.1 Demonstrate the use of the Index of Orthodontic Treatment Need (IOTN)

12.2 Demonstrate the use of the Peer Assessment Rating (PAR)

12.3 Understand the relevance of prioritising treatment

12.4 Describe and be able to use methods of assessing outcomes of treatment

12.5 Understand the complexity of treatment and the hierarchy of treatment providers

The syllabus for the Certificate in Orthodontic Nursing is reproduced by kind permission of the NEBDN (requested and granted in 2019). Detailed information on all courses is available from NEBDN (see Useful contacts section for how to access this information).

For many orthodontic nurses, the Certificate in Orthodontic Nursing is a logical progression in their career pathway. For some it is a means to an end, for others it is a gateway to their next step, to become an orthodontic therapist (see Chapter 26).

In addition to the Certificate of Orthodontic Nursing, other courses run for post-registration qualifications include

- Certificate in Oral Health
- Certificate in Dental Sedation Nursing
- Certificate in Special Needs Nursing
- Certificate in Dental Radiography
- Application of Topical Fluoride and Fissure Sealant.

CERTIFICATE IN ORTHODONTIC NURSING

This information is also reproduced by kind permission of NEBDN. The NEBDN wishes to point out that it is keen to encourage all students to use a variety of sources for their learning.

Orthodontic nurses with appropriate training now carry out extended duties including taking dental impressions, clinical photographs and dental radiography. The *Orthodontic Specialist Group* (OSG), a group within the British Orthodontic Society, has established an in-house training resource that allows the nurses to receive training.

There are (as of spring 2019) training modules available for taking impressions and clinical photography.

MODULE IN THE TAKING OF IMPRESSIONS

Practical session notes: Unit 1

When taking dental impressions, the clinician will need to consider factors that will affect the quality of the impression:

- patient communication
- suitable tray selection
- quality of the mix and consistency of impression material
- clinical technique and patient preparation.

Patient communication

- always gain consent before proceeding:
  - **implied consent:** patient sits in the chair, implying that they are ready to proceed
  - **informed consent:** patient is informed of the procedure and gives consent
  - **verbal consent:** patient gives consent by word.
- always explain the procedure to the patient (and accompanying parent or carer).
- always observe the patient throughout the procedure and be aware of signs of emotional or physical anxiety.
- reassure the anxious patient.

Suitable tray selection
Impression trays can vary depending on clinical procedure.

- look in the patient's mouth
- select tray.
- try in the patient's mouth and make sure it:
  - covers the teeth
  - extends comfortably into the sulci
  - does not over- or under-extend.

Quality of impression mix

There are many factors to consider when mixing alginate impression material.

- always check the expiry date of impression material.
- always ensure that the powder is stored in an airtight container.
- shake and invert the powder before dispensing.
- use correct scoop, overloading and levelling off with a mixing spatula.
- use correct powder-to-water ratio (optimum temperature 21°C).
- mix to a smooth creamy consistency with no air bubbles. Use manufacturer's time guidelines on mixing, working and setting times.

Technique of clinician and patient preparation

- the patient can be upright or supine: always move the chair so that the patient is in the best position for you to proceed. This ensures that the clinician is not stooping or overstretched when taking the impression.
- ensure correct loading of tray: hold handle and load tray so that all areas needed are covered. Turn tray over and check that there are no air bubbles.
- manipulation of the loaded tray (practical demonstration and lesson).

Silicones and polyethers

The impression material usually comes in two components:

- base
- catalyst.

These are mixed together by hand, ensuring both components are evenly distributed, and formed into a sausage and loaded into the tray. Lighter-bodied silicones and polyethers are often distributed using a gun to mix the base and catalyst together.

Practical session notes: Unit 2

Preparation of patient

- inform patient of procedure
- obtain informed consent
- advise patient.

Positioning patient

- patient can be either upright or supine.
- make sure chair is in the correct position for the clinician to prevent straining or over-reaching.

Correct loading of alginate in tray

- hold tray by handle.
- place sufficient alginate material to cover tray edges.

- do not overfill.
- turn tray over to ensure the holes are filled; if not, then push the alginate in further using spatula to eliminate air bubbles.
- smooth off excess material.

Position of clinician

- if the patient is upright, stand in front of the patient for the lower and behind for the upper arch.
- if supine, sit behind the patient for both arches.

Manipulation of loaded tray

Insertion in the mouth

- use this method when trying the trays in for size:
  - ask the patient to open their mouth.
  - gently retract lips and cheeks.
  - slide tray over the teeth, one side first then the other.
  - in the lower arch, ask the patient to curl tongue to the back of the mouth.

Seating the tray

- in the lower arch, as the loaded tray is over the teeth, gently press the loaded tray down onto the anterior teeth first and then apply pressure all the way round whilst holding the lips and cheeks away from the tray.
- in the upper arch, gently press the loaded tray buccally before applying even pressure all the way round.
- ensure tray is fully seated into the sulci and not traumatic to the soft tissue.
- muscle trim.

Setting of material

- do not move tray whilst setting.
- maintain firm pressure on the body of the tray.
- avoid dragging the impression material.
- check that material is set and then leave a little longer to ensure the material is fully set throughout the impression.

Removal from the mouth

- do not apply pressure on the tray handle.
- free seal in the buccal sulci bilaterally.
- free anteriorly.
- lift out vertically.
- twist impression tray to remove from the mouth.
- rinse and disinfect impression.

Ideal features of the dental impression

- all the surfaces of the erupted teeth.
- fully extended into the labial and buccal sulcus to ensure that when impression is cast the model shows all the teeth and the supporting alveolus.
- palatal vault as far as the distal surfaces of the first molars.

Recording the occlusion (bite)

- soften pink wax wafer.
- make into a horseshoe shape.
- place on the occlusal surface of the teeth.
- buccal teeth in centric occlusion.
- remove, cool and disinfect.

Recording orthodontic occlusion for functional orthodontic appliance

This can only be carried out by an orthodontist, orthodontic therapist or a general dental practitioner (GDP).

Errors that occur during the taking of impressions

These can occur because of:

- errors in the mixing of the dental impression material
- errors in positioning of the impression tray
- the early removal of the impression tray
- patient anxiety (pulling tray out, strong gag reflex, frightened)
- inexperience.

MODULE IN CLINICAL PHOTOGRAPHY

This course is made up of four main modules:

- Clinical Photographs – The Gold Standard by J. Sandler and A. Williams
- Clinical Photography in Orthodontic Practice Environment, Part 1
- Clinical Photography in Orthodontic Practice Environment, Part 2
- Photograph Protocol as a PowerPoint presentation with information and photographs.

For further information and details of both these courses, please go to the British Orthodontic Society website at http://bos.org.uk and access nurse education courses. Both syllabuses are reproduced by kind permission of the British Orthodontic Society.

CERTIFICATE IN ORTHODONTIC NURSING

Chapter 26

Orthodontic therapists

For the orthodontic dental nurse who has taken the Certificate in Orthodontic Dental Nursing and wishes to further expand their ongoing professional development, the next logical step could be to apply for enrolment on a course to become an orthodontic therapist.

The orthodontic therapy courses began in 2007 and from the beginning there was a great deal of interest in them. While some of the training is provided at training centres, every student works under the supervision of a dedicated trainer. The trainers have themselves been trained to undertake this. The trainer will be a specialist orthodontist who works in either secondary care (a hospital department or a community clinic) or in primary care in a specialist practice.

Courses follow a modular format. At the start of the course, the first 8 weeks will contain the core teaching in an alternate weekly pattern.

- week 1: they are based at their training centre.
- week 2: they are in their own training unit or training practice.

This alternate weekly pattern continues until the student has undergone four 5-day weeks of training until 20 days of core training are completed. To be successful the candidate must be given sufficient free time to attend the core teaching.

Competition for places is keen. Applications are taken from:

- dental nurses
- dental hygienists
- dental therapists
- dental technicians.

All need to be registered with the General Dental Council (GDC) and have experience of working full time (or the equivalent) for at least a year post qualification.

The training for dental technicians is different: they have to be able to demonstrate that they have been on a foundation course to understand the clinical and management side of working with patients in a dental surgery. They must also be able to show knowledge of cross-infection, etc.

Basic Guide to Orthodontic Dental Nursing, Second Edition. Fiona Grist.
© 2020 John Wiley & Sons Ltd. Published 2020 by John Wiley & Sons Ltd.

The orthodontic therapist works under the prescription of a dentist. Only the dentist can:

- decide on a treatment plan
- make a diagnosis of disease
- adjust or activate an archwire.

THE SYLLABUS FOR ORTHODONTIC THERAPY

Biomedical sciences and oral biology

- have the knowledge and understanding of those aspects of the biomedical sciences, oral physiology and craniofacial, oral and dental anatomy that are significant in the management of patients.
- be familiar with those aspects of general anatomy, physiology and biochemistry relevant to orthodontic therapy.

Medical emergencies

- be competent at carrying out resuscitation techniques.
- have knowledge of how to identify medical emergencies and provide immediate management of anaphylactic reaction, hypoglycaemia, upper respiratory obstruction, cardiac arrest, fits, vasovagal attack, inhalation or ingestion of foreign bodies, or haemorrhage.
- be familiar with the principles of first aid.

Dental biomaterials science

- be competent in the correct selection and manipulation of the dental biomaterials used by orthodontic therapists.
- have knowledge of the science that underpins the dental biomaterials used by the orthodontic therapist.
- have knowledge of the limitations of such dental biomaterials.
- be familiar with those aspects of biomaterials safety that relate to the work of the orthodontic therapist.

Pain and anxiety control

- be competent at managing fear and anxiety with behavioural techniques and empathise with patients in stressful situations.
- be familiar with the manifestations of anxiety and pain, and the various methods available for their management control.

Human disease

- have knowledge of the scientific principles of sterilisation, disinfection and antisepsis.
- be familiar with the implications of a positive medical history and the main medical disorders that may affect the provision of orthodontic treatment.

ORTHODONTIC THERAPISTS

Health and safety and infection control

- be competent at implementing and performing satisfactory infection control and preventing physical, chemical and microbiological contamination in the clinic and the laboratory.
- be competent at arranging and using the working clinical and laboratory environment in the most safe and efficient manner.
- have knowledge of health and safety legislation as it affects clinical and laboratory practice.

Comprehensive oral care

- be competent at working with other members of the dental team.
- be competent at interpreting and working to an orthodontic care plan or prescription.
- have knowledge of the role of the orthodontic therapist within the framework of the dental team.
- have knowledge of when to refer the patient to a dentist, where treatment is beyond the training or experience of the orthodontic therapist.
- be familiar with the organisation of the orthodontic services within the UK.

Behavioural sciences, communication skills and health informatics

- be competent at using the latest information technology.
- be competent at communication with patients, their families and carers, other members of the dental team and other healthcare professionals.
- have knowledge of managing patients from different social and ethnic backgrounds.
- have knowledge of working as part of the dental team.
- be familiar with the social and psychological issues relevant to the care of patients.

Law, ethics and professionalism

- be competent at maintaining full and accurate clinical records.
- have knowledge of responsibilities of consent, duty of care and confidentiality.
- have knowledge of patients' rights and how to handle complaints.
- have knowledge of the range of skills of other members of the dental team.
- have knowledge of the regulatory functions of the GDC.
- have knowledge of their responsibilities in relation to the referral of patients.
- be familiar with the legal and ethical obligations of registered members of the dental team.
- be familiar with the obligation to practice in the best interests of the patient at all times.
- be familiar with the need for lifelong learning and professional development.
- be familiar with the law as it applies to records.

THE SYLLABUS FOR CLINICAL ORTHODONTICS

Clinical records

- be competent at taking intra-oral and extra-oral photographs of patients, and photographs of models and radiographs.
- be competent at taking dental impressions.
- be competent at taking and checking occlusal records, including gnathological facebow readings.
- be competent at casting, basing and trimming orthodontic models.
- be competent at producing a cephalometric analysis of a skull radiograph by contemporary methods.

Principles of orthodontics

- have knowledge of the features of normal and ideal occlusion.
- have knowledge of the classification of malocclusion.
- have knowledge of the principles of tooth movement, force application and anchorage.
- have knowledge of common orthodontic appliance systems and their mechanical principles.
- be familiar with the aetiology of malocclusion.
- be familiar with the limitations of orthodontic treatment.
- be familiar with the potential risks and benefits of orthodontic treatment, including iatrogenic damage.

Orthodontic instruments

- be competent at identifying and selecting appropriate instruments for the task to be carried out.
- be competent at using equipment and instruments safely.
- be competent at maintaining instruments.

Removable appliance placement

- be competent at inserting passive removable appliances.
- be competent at inserting active removable appliances previously adjusted by a dentist.
- be competent at fitting orthodontic headgear.
- be competent at fitting orthodontic facebows having been previously adjusted by a dentist.
- be competent at measuring elastic headgear forces.

Fixed appliance placement

- be competent at placing and removing orthodontic separators.
- be competent at identifying and selecting orthodontic bands appropriate for the patient.

ORTHODONTIC THERAPISTS

- be competent at placing, adapting and cementing bands to achieve an ideal fit.
- be competent at identifying attachments appropriate for individual teeth.
- be competent at cleaning and preparing the tooth surface for orthodontic bonding.
- be competent at using orthodontic adhesives and cements.
- be competent at placing attachments, including bonded retainers, onto the teeth in the correct position.
- be competent at preparing archwires.
- be competent at inserting and ligating archwires and archwire auxiliaries.
- be competent at ligating groups of teeth together.
- be familiar with the technique of welding attachments to bands.

Fixed appliance removal

- be competent at releasing and removing ligatures.
- be competent at removing archwires and archwire auxiliaries.
- be competent at removing cemented and bonded attachments.
- be competent at differentiating between dental tissues, dental deposits and cement residues from the teeth.
- be competent at supragingival cleaning and polishing of the teeth using both powered and manual instrumentation, and at stain removal and prophylaxis where directly relevant to orthodontic treatment.

Orthodontic emergency care

- be competent at identifying damaged and distorted orthodontic appliances.
- be competent at taking limited action to relieve pain and make an appliance safe in the absence of a dentist.
- be competent at identifying when a situation is beyond the orthodontic therapist's expertise and requires the patient to be seen by a dentist.
- have knowledge of the need to arrange early attention by a dentist following the emergency treatment.

In the future this list may broaden still further to include:

- removing sutures on the instruction of a dentist
- applying topical fluoride varnish as indicated by the dentist
- repairing the acrylic components on removable orthodontic appliances
- measuring and recording gingival indices and plaque indices.

However, some procedures are reserved for dentists, dental therapists and dental hygienists. These include:

- giving local anaesthetics
- performing deep (subgingival) scaling
- fitting temporary dressings
- re-cementing crowns or bridges.

The syllabus described in this chapter is reproduced by kind permission of the General Dental Council (accessed in 2019). The British Orthodontic Society has also published

ORTHODONTIC THERAPISTS

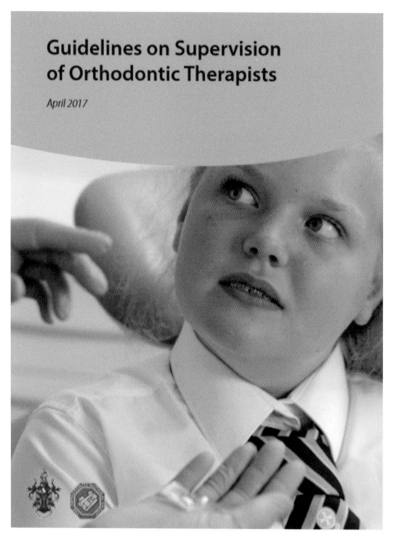

Figure 26.1 Guidelines on the supervision of orthodontic therapists. Source: Reproduced by kind permission of the British Orthodontic Society.

Guidelines on the Supervision of Orthodontic Therapists (Figure 26.1), which can be accessed at www.bos.org.uk/Portals/0/Public/docs/General%20Guidance/GuidelinesonSu pervisionofOrthodonticTherapistsApril2017.pdf

Chapter 27

The Orthodontic National Group for Dental Nurses and Therapists

In June 1994, the Orthodontic National Group (ONG) was formed as an independent specialist group for dental nurses in the UK and Ireland. From its initial meeting the aims and objectives were clear.

AIMS

To act on behalf of all Orthodontic Dental Nurses and subsequently Therapists to advance high standards by developing and expanding their roles under 'Dental Care Professionals'.

OBJECTIVES

- to develop the Orthodontic Dental Nurses and Therapist roles within the Specialist Group.
- to provide continuing professional education with at least bi-annual study days.
- to keep the membership informed by means of Newsletters and Web Site.
- to recommend to the General Dental Council (GDC) changes needed in legislation.
- to liaise with relevant professional bodies to promote the status of:
  - Orthodontic Dental Nurses and Therapists
  - to manage the Group's finances to achieve its objectives
  - to plan for the future.

From the onset the goal was to create career pathways for dental nurses that would provide them with continuing professional development (CPD), extended duties and recognition as dental care professionals (DCPs).

The Group has a distinctive badge and logo, an orthodontic bracket (Figure 27.1). The bracket has a yellow line filling the bracket slot recognises the affiliation with dental nursing.

Basic Guide to Orthodontic Dental Nursing, Second Edition. Fiona Grist.
© 2020 John Wiley & Sons Ltd. Published 2020 by John Wiley & Sons Ltd.

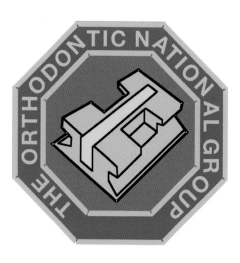

Figure 27.1 ONG logo. Source: Reproduced by kind permission of Orthodontic National Group.

THE ORTHODONTIC NATIONAL GROUP

In 2005, the title of the Group name was amended to Orthodontic Nurses and Therapists to encompass these rapidly developing roles as DCPs.

A prime objective has always been to develop the role of orthodontic dental nurses and therapists within the specialists group. The curriculum for the Orthodontic Therapist course had input from the ONG and it was due in part to their direct representation to the GDC that the title Orthodontic Therapist was accepted.

The ONG was also represented on the group that worked on the curriculum for the now well-established post-qualification Certificate in Orthodontic Nursing.

In order to achieve this, the Group has always maintained a small and efficient elected Committee. All of them are busy working orthodontic nurses and therapists so are able to relate to issues and difficulties that their colleagues might face.

STRUCTURE OF THE GROUP

The Committee meets every quarter and holds its Annual General Meeting at the British Orthodontic Conference, which is usually held in September. In recent years, in addition to the Committee, the post of President has been added. The Group has been represented at the GDC, the British Dental Association and the Royal Colleges.

EDUCATION

The ONG has aimed to provide a focus for orthodontic education and development. As part of the British Orthodontic Conference, the nurses have parallel programmes. The British Orthodontic Society (BOS) has invited the ONG to submit suggested topics and speakers for this. The Nurse and Therapist programmes prove very popular. Each year the number of delegates exceeds 400, making it significantly the largest meeting of orthodontic nurses and therapists in the country.

Annual registration with the GDC for orthodontic dental nurses and orthodontic therapists carries with it an expectation that they will maintain their level of CPD. Outlines for these are monitored to amend and update. Using their GDC number, a nurse or therapist can get the latest current information from the GDC website. The GDC also produce learning outcomes – a framework of skills, knowledge and abilities that should be in place at the end of qualifying training. This can be accessed at https://www.gdc-uk.org/professionals/education

JOURNAL

From the outset in 1994, as part of its commitment to education, the Group published a journal for its members. The journal has a strong bias towards clinical topics, with a high educational content. Also included are articles written for and by dental nurses and therapists that aim to keep members abreast of current policies, technical data and recent changes to legislation. The format and name of the newsletter changed in 2003 to become *ONG News*.

LINKS WITH THE BRITISH ORTHODONTIC SOCIETY

In 1997, the ONG became an affiliated organisation of the BOS, which had for many years been encouraging the team approach within the specialty. Many orthodontists actively encourage their nurses to go on courses, to Conference, provide them with CPD and financially support their development. The BOS not only encourages the Nurses and Therapists Days, but also allows them access to the lectures on the scientific programme in the main auditorium on the other days. Throughout the year they also welcome and encourage attendance at the meetings of the many groups that make up the society. As part of the annual subscription, in addition to *ONG News*, members also receive *BOS News* and *Bulletin of Clinical Effectiveness*.

THE FUTURE

The ONG continues to liaise on behalf of its members with the orthodontic and wider dental community, valuing professionalism both from itself and its members. It is not just in the field of orthodontics that nurses and therapists benefit, as the ONG continues to focus on assistance and guidance for their members across a wide variety of areas.

THE ORTHODONTIC NATIONAL GROUP

CONTACT DETAILS

The Orthodontic National Group for Dental Nurses and Therapists
12 Bridewell Place
London EC4V 6AP
Email: ann.wright@bos.org.uk (membership enquiries)
ONG911@outlook.com
Telephone: 020 7353 8680
Website: www.orthodontic-ong.org

Other groups also work for and on behalf of dental nurses. Their contact details are:

British Association of Dental Nurses (BADN)
Room 200
Hillhouse International Site
Fleetwood Road North
Thornton-Cleveleys FY5 4QD
Telephone: 01253 338360
Website: www.badn.org.uk

Society of British Dental Nurses
21 Waterloo Place
Leamington Spa CV32 5LA
Telephone: 07824 703741, 01530 224648
Email: info@sbdn.org.uk
Website: https://sbdn.org.uk/

THE ORTHODONTIC NATIONAL GROUP

Useful contacts

British Orthodontic Society (BOS)

12, Bridewell Place
London EC4V 6AP
Email: ann.wright@bos.org.uk
Telephone: 020 7353 8680
Fax: 020 7353 8682
Website: www.bos.org.uk

General Dental Council (GDC)

37 Wimpole Street
London W1G 8DQ
Email: dcp@gdc-uk.org
Telephone: 020 7887 3800
Fax: 020 7224 3294
Website: www.gdc-uk.org

British Dental Association (BDA)

64 Wimpole Street
London W1G 8YS
Email: enquiries@bda.org
Telephone: 020 7935 0875
Fax: 020 7487 5232
Website: www.bda.org

Orthodontic National Group for Dental Nurses and Therapists (ONG)

12 Bridewell Place
London EC4V 6AP
Email: ann.wright@bos.org.uk (membership enquiries)
ONG911@outlook.com
Telephone: 020 7353 8680
Website: www.orthodontic-ong.org

Basic Guide to Orthodontic Dental Nursing, Second Edition. Fiona Grist.
© 2020 John Wiley & Sons Ltd. Published 2020 by John Wiley & Sons Ltd.

British Association of Dental Nurses (BADN)

PO Box 4
Room 200
Hillhouse International Business Centre
Thornton-Cleveleys FY5 4QD
Email: editor@badn.org.uk
Telephone: 01253 338360
Website: www.badn.org.uk

Society of British Dental Nurses (SBDN)

21 Waterloo Place
Leamington Spa CV32 SLA
Email: info@sbdn.org.uk
Telephone: 07824 703704
Website: www.sbdn.org.uk

National Examining Board for Dental Nurses (NEBDN)

First Floor
Quayside Court
Chain Caul Way
Preston PR2 2ZP
Email: info@nebn.org
Telephone: 01772 429917
Website: www.nebn.org

Companies supplying orthodontic equipment and sundries

American Orthodontics
Riverside House
2a Mill Road
Marlow SL7 1PX
Email: ortho@americanorthodontics.co.uk
Telephone: 01628 477921
Website: www.americanortho.com

DB Orthodontics
Unit 6, Ryefield Way, Silden, Keighley, BD20 OEF
Email: sales@dbortho.com
Telephone: 01535 656999
Website: www.dbortho.com

Forestadent
Unit 1
Crossinglands Business Park
Salford Road
Aspley Guise MK17 8HZ
Email: info@forestadent.co.uk
Telephone: 01908 227851
Website: www.forestadent.co.uk

3M Unitek
Charnwood Campus
10 Bakewell Road
Loughborough LE11 5RD
Email: 3MUnitek@mmm.com
Telephone: 0845 873 4066
Website: www.3MUnitek.com

Ortho-Care (UK) Ltd
1 Riverside Estate
Saltaire BD17 7DR
Email: info@orthocare.co.uk
Telephone: 01274 533233
Website: www.orthocare.co.uk

Precision Orthodontics Ltd
Ashley House
58–60 Ashley Road
Hampton TW12 2HU
Email: post@percsisionorthodontics.com
Telephone: 0208 979 9493
Website: www.precisionorthodontics.com

The Dental Directory
6 Perry Way
Witham CM8 3SX
Email: sales@dental-directory.co.uk
Telephone: 01376 391100
Website: www.dental-directory.co.uk

TOC
The Old Church
Collins Street
Avonmouth Village
Bristol BS11 9JJ
Email: info@tocdental.com
Website: www.tocdental.com

USEFUL CONTACTS

T P Orthodontics
Fountain Court
12 Bruntcliffe Way
Morley
Leeds LS27 0JG
Email: tpeng@tportho.com
Telephone: 0113 2539192
Website: www.tportho.com

Optident Ltd
International Development Centre
Valley Drive
Ilkley LS29 8PD
Email: sales@optident.co.uk
Telephone: 01943 605050
Website: www.optident.co.uk

This is merely a guide to some of the many companies that specialise in orthodontic equipment and supplies.

Glossary

Abfraction – wear caused by tooth being too high on the bite

Abrasion – wear caused by repeated action, i.e. excessive tooth brushing

Aesthetic component – part of the Index of Orthodontic Treatment Need, relates to degree of malocclusion judged by appearance

Aesthetic plane – line used in tracing lateral cephelometric radiographs, from the soft tissue tip of the nose to the soft tissue tip of the chin

Alginate – a type of material used in taking orthodontic impressions

Aligner – clear plastic splints, which are worn to align teeth; 'often' several used in a course of treatment

Alveolar bone graft – addition of bone when it is lacking, e.g. cleft and implant patients

Alveolar ridge – part of mouth that carries the teeth

Anchorage – point from which force is applied

Angle's classification – classification of malocclusion based on the relationship between the upper and lower first molars

Ankylosis – condition where the root is fused to the bone (often as a result of trauma); it is an anatomical fusion between the alveolar bone and the cementum and cannot be moved orthodontically

Anodontia – absence of teeth

Anterior – at the front of the mouth, opposite of posterior

Anterior open bite – where there is no contact when front teeth bite together

Anti-habit appliances – a fixed or removable appliance with built-in wire that acts as deterrent to thumb or finger sucking

Apical – relating to the apex (tip) of the tooth root

Archwire – wire which fits into the attached component of fixed appliance

Assessment – an orthodontic examination of a patient's malocclusion

Attrition – tooth wear caused by repeated tooth onto tooth friction, e.g. bruxism (grinding of teeth, especially at night)

Ball end clasp – part of a removable appliance fitting into tooth undercuts to aid retention of the appliance

Banding – fitting molar bands

Begg retainer – upper acrylic retainer with labial bow but no Adams cribs

Bimaxillary – both maxilla and mandible

Bite-raising appliance – appliance with acrylic over the occlusal surfaces to disengage the occlusion

Basic Guide to Orthodontic Dental Nursing, Second Edition. Fiona Grist.
© 2020 John Wiley & Sons Ltd. Published 2020 by John Wiley & Sons Ltd.

Bonded retainer – wire permanently fixed to teeth to stop them moving (nearly always lingual surface)

Bonding – fixing attachments directly to the tooth surface (brackets, cleats, etc.)

Bone harvesting – taking bone from one part of the body for use elsewhere

Brace – a commonly used term for an orthodontic appliance

Bruxism – grinding together of teeth, often in sleep

Buccal – relating to the cheek-facing surface of the tooth

Buccal segment – the first premolar to the last molar in a quadrant

Buccal sulcus – space between the teeth and alveolar bone and the cheek

Caries – dental decay

Casting – making a model of the teeth from an impression

Centre line – vertical line running between the upper and the lower central incisors

Centric occlusion – the occlusion of the teeth when they fully touch together from an open mouth position without displacing

Cephalometric analysis – results of measurements made on a cephalometric radiograph either using manual tracing or computer software

Cephalometric radiograph – a true side-view radiograph of the skull and face showing the relationship between the teeth and relative facial bones

Cervical strap – strap used with extra-oral traction which is placed around the back of the neck, similar function to a head cap

Cheek retractor – plastic device to keep the lips and cheeks from coming into contact with the teeth

Cingulum pad – part of the palatal aspect of upper incisor crown, towards the cervical

Clasp – wire used on a removable appliance to give retention

Class I – an occlusion which is normal but with tooth irregularities

Class II – a malocclusion where the upper teeth are forward in relation to the lowers; there are two divisions of this class

Class III – a malocclusion where the lower incisor teeth bite either edge to edge or in front of the upper incisor teeth

Cleats – hook-shaped attachment which can be bonded to teeth or welded to bands

Cleft lip – where there is a congenital gap or notch in the upper lip/alveolus

Cleft palate – where there has been incomplete midline fusion of the palate before birth

Clinical crown – the part of the crown that is visible, e.g. that can be used for orthodontic attachments as opposed to the anatomical crown

Coil – can be supplied open or closed, usually comes on spools, hollow coiled wire which is put over an archwire to either push open a space or prevent a space from closing

Congenital defect – one present before birth

Consultation – appointment between patient and orthodontist to assess and discuss treatment options

Crossbite – where the lower teeth are incorrectly biting outside the upper teeth; can be applicable to buccal segment (posterior) or anterior teeth

Crowding – not enough space in the dental arch to accommodate the teeth in good alignment

Curing light – ultraviolet light used to 'set' dental adhesives and cements

Debanding – removal of bands

Debonding – removal of brackets

Decalcification – loss of hard (mineralised) dental tissue through acid attack

Deciduous dentition – first teeth, which are lost, also called primary, milk or baby teeth, 20 in total; early loss can affect eruption and positioning of permanent teeth

Decontamination – cleaning of instruments prior to sterilisation

Dens-in-dente – a malformation; literally a 'tooth within a tooth'

Dental age – apparent age of the dentition, which may not be the same as the chronological age of the patient

Dental arch – the position and form of the teeth in the upper and lower jaws

Dental health component – part of the Index of Orthodontic Treatment Need, deals with obvious clinical problems, such as crossbites, overjets, rotations, etc.

Deviation – when the mandible deflects in its path of closure

Diastema – gap between teeth, commonly upper central incisors

Digit sucking – thumb or finger sucking habit

Displacement – when the mandible's path of closure is deviated because there is an occlusal obstruction initially

Distraction osteogenesis – lengthening of bones by a rapid expansion system following surgical cuts in the bone

Ectopic canine – canine tooth that has been deflected from its natural path of eruption and has gone off course

Enamel – mineralised hard outer surface of the anatomical crown of both deciduous and permanent teeth

Erosion – where there is damage to the tooth from acid attack, especially by 'sugar-free' and carbonated drinks

Eruption pattern – the timing of the eruption of deciduous and permanent teeth

Essix appliance – clear vacuum-formed thermoplastic retainer, which looks like a thin gum shield and is usually worn at night

Expansion screws – screws which are turned to open and expand

Extra-oral – not in the mouth

Extra-oral anchorage – use of the back of the head or neck as anchor points

Facebow – an inner and outer bow welded together, used in extra-oral traction; the inner bow fits into the buccal tubes on a removable or fixed appliance

Fixed appliance – appliance that is fixed to the teeth and cannot be removed by the patient

Fixed retainer – retainer that is fixed to the teeth and cannot be removed by the patient

Fluoride – element found naturally in water which impedes caries; often added to water supply, toothpaste and mouthwash

Frankfort plane – used in assessment and when tracing lateral cephalometric radiographs; a horizontal plane which is reckoned to be parallel with the ground when humans walk upright

Frenectomy – removal of the frenum

Frenum – web of fleshy tissue in both maxilla and mandible notably in the midline between the lips and the gingivae

Functional appliance – type of appliance, removable or fixed, that helps to reduce increased overjets and encourage better development of the mandible

Genioplasty – surgical repositioning of the chin

Gingiva – the gum around a tooth

Gingivitis – inflammation of the gums, which can be localised and may be chronic or acute

Growth spurt – a child's period of rapid growth, usually during puberty; helpful when using functional appliances

Hawley retainer – removable retainer made of acrylic and wire components

Headgear – consists of a cervical or head band and a facebow which fits onto either fixed tubes on bands or a removable appliance in the mouth

Hypodontia – congenitally missing tooth or teeth

Hypoplastic – poorly formed, e.g. enamel defects

ICON (Index of Complexity, Outcome and Need) – an assessment Index measuring the severity of malocclusion and treatment complexity

Impaction – when the normal process of tooth eruption has not occurred because there is a resistance to it, e.g. wisdom tooth impacted into second molars

Impression – imprint, using a soft material that sets; when cast it gives a reproduction; alginate is most commonly used in orthodontics

Incisor relationship – how the upper and lower incisors relate in occlusion

Index of Orthodontic Treatment Need (IOTN) – index used for standardising the criteria of orthodontic need

Infra-occlusion – tooth or teeth at a lower level than the occlusal plane

Interproximal reduction – making space between the contact points of teeth using a fine bur, disc or blade to reduce the thickness of proximal enamel

Intramaxillary traction – tooth movement occasioned by force from a point in the same dental arch

Intra-oral – inside the mouth

Intrusion – moving teeth orthodontically into the alveolar bone

Invagination – an abnormal indentation in the crown of a tooth

Kesling set-up – from a cast of the teeth, individual plaster teeth are cut off and repositioned on the model, to a prescription

Labial bow – wire bow over the 'front' of the anterior teeth

Labial segment – incisor teeth (often includes the canines)

Leaflets – information about treatment and care

Ligature – soft wire, e.g. used to tie in archwires

Lingual arch – a metal wire formed to the lingual outline of the lower arch

Lingual archwires – of various alloys, designed for use in the lingual technique

Lingual orthodontics – treatment where the brackets are fixed onto the inside of the teeth, the tongue side

Lip line – the position of the upper lip outline in relation to the upper incisor teeth

Lip trap – when the lower lip gets trapped behind the upper front teeth

Macrodont – larger than normal tooth

Malocclusion – where there is an incorrect relationship between the dental arches and/or the teeth

Mandible – the lower jaw

Mandibular plane – used in tracing lateral cephalometric radiographs; line of the lower border of the mandible

Masel safety strap – strap which is placed over the external J hooks on a facebow to give extra security

Maxilla – the upper jaw

Maxillary plane – used in tracing lateral cephalometric radiographs; a line between the posterior and anterior borders of the hard palate

Mesiodens – a supernumerary tooth in the midline between the upper incisors

Microdont – smaller than normal tooth

Microdontia – abnormally small teeth

Midline Dental – upper and lower dental arches

       Facial – vertical line of face

Mini screws – temporary anchorage devices (TADs)

Model box – where patient's models are stored; each patient has their own individual box

Molar relationship – relationship mesio-distally of the occlusion of the first molars

Mouthguard – semi-flexible appliance used to protect teeth when playing contact sports

Nickel titanium (NiTi) – alloy material from which some archwires are made

Obstructive sleep apnoea (OSA) – condition where patient has incomplete sleep pattern, can sometimes be woken by feelings of not breathing and choking

Occlusal plane – used when tracing lateral cephelometric radiographs; a line between the teeth in occlusion

Occlusal rest – a wire component of a removable appliance which lies over the occlusal surface of a molar

Occlusion – the relation in contact between the upper and lower dental arches

Odontome – abnormal mass of dental tissue

Oligodontia – several congenitally missing teeth

Open bite – when opposing teeth are not biting together in occlusion

Oral hygiene – maintaining a clean and healthy mouth

Oral surgery – surgery relating to the mouth, both skeletal, dental, and soft tissue

Orthodontist – one who practices orthodontics; usually speciality trained and registered

Orthognathic surgery – surgery to the jaw(s) to correct malrelationship

Orthopantomograph (OPT) – radiograph taken as scan view of all the teeth; X-ray tube moves around the patient's head

Osteogenesis – *see* distraction osteogenesis

Osteotomy – surgical procedure to correct skeletal-related malocclusion

Overbite – when the upper front teeth overlap the lower teeth vertically

Overjet – how much the upper front teeth protrude or retrude horizontally in relation to the lower teeth

Palatal arch – wire that spans the palate, soldered to bands cemented to the molars

Palate – roof of the mouth; there is a hard and a soft palate with the soft posterior to the hard

PAR (Peer Assessment Rating) – an occlusal index to measure on study models the degree of improvement after orthodontic treatment

Peg-shaped – misshapen, usually conical, tooth crown

Periodontal – relating to the supporting tissues of the teeth

Permanent dentition – the adult quota of 32 teeth: 8 incisors, 4 canines, 8 premolars and 12 molars

Photographic mirrors – palatal, buccal or lingual mirrors for intra-oral photography

Piercing – oral jewellery, lip, cheek and tongue studs or hoops

Plaque – a soft clear substance made from saliva and bacteria

Porcelain primer – used on porcelain crown and veneers before attaching brackets

Positioners – removable 'retaining' appliances that are also actively moving certain teeth

Posterior – at the back, opposite of anterior

Posterior open bite – where teeth do not bite together towards the back of the mouth

Posturing habit – bringing the lower jaw forwards in order to close the lips

Proclined – angled forwards

Quad helix – upper fixed appliance to widen arch; *quad* means four, *helix* means circle

Radiograph – image made using X-rays

Rapid maxillary expansion (RME) – appliance cemented onto teeth, with an expansion screw in palate, turned by patient

Referral – request from a dentist for a specialist consultation

Relapse – the occlusion returning to pre-treatment irregularities

Removable appliance – appliance that can be taken in and out of the mouth by the patient

Retainer – an inactive appliance that holds teeth in position to prevent relapse; can be removable or fixed

Retention – maintaining corrected teeth in their corrected positions

Retroclined – angled backwards

Reverse pull headgear – system which aims to bring the maxillary arch forward; used in Class lll cases

Roberts retractor – active removable appliance with a labial bow which has high loops built into it

Root resorption – when the root becomes shorter; sometimes occurs as a side effect of orthodontic treatment; can also be pathological

Rotation – when a tooth is twisted from the correct position

Scissor bite – when upper buccal segment teeth bite totally outside lowers

Screws – can be used for expansion; used as temporary anchorage devices (mini screws)

Self-ligating brackets – brackets with an 'arm' that can open and close over the wire slot; avoids need for O-rings and ligatures

Separating pliers – pliers used for placing separating rings, also known as force separating pliers

Separating springs – used when rubber separating rings will not slip through contact points, inserted using Weingart or spring-forming pliers

Separators – devices placed between the teeth to open space prior to fitting bands

Sharps box – container for all used or unwanted metal, wires, bands, etc.

Skeletal pattern – maxilla and mandible relationship, usually in antero-posterior plane

Sleep apnoea – disruption of normal sleep rhythm and often accompanied by snoring and an interrupted breathing pattern

Southend clasp – clasp used on removable appliances; positioned at the cervical margin of upper centrals

Space maintainer – appliance that keeps space open in a dental arch

Spacing – natural gaps between teeth in the same dental arch

Speech and language therapist (SALT) – therapist who helps with speech, which is often an issue for patients with clefts

Spider screws – type of temporary anchorage device

Springs – used in both removable and fixed appliances to move teeth

Stability – ability of teeth to remain in their corrected position after orthodontic treatment

Sterilisation – to make sterile

Stripping – removing enamel mesially and distally to provide space

Study models – casts used as records

Submerged – tooth sinking back below the occlusal level into the gum

Supernumerary tooth – an additional tooth, more than usual; often remains unerupted

T spring – spring used on removable appliances, shaped like the letter T

Temporary anchorage device (TAD) – small screw which can be placed directly into the alveolar bone for a short time and are easily removed; they provide an anchorage point

Temporo-mandibular joint (TMJ) – complex joint where the mandible opens and closes (the condyles can be felt moving by your the ears when you open and close your mouth)

Tongue studs – studs piercing the tongue

Tongue thrust – an involuntary habit; a strong movement which can cause problems with positions of dental arches and speech

Tooth wear – results of tooth surface loss

Torque – force to correct the inclination of teeth labio-lingually/bucco-lingually

Tracing – measurements from a lateral cephalometric tracing

Traction – tension, pulling

Transposition – when position of teeth is interchanged, an abnormality

Trauma – injury

Traumatic occlusion – occlusion that is causing self-damage

Treatment plan – choice of treatment based on assessment

Twin blocks – functional appliance consisting of upper and lower removable appliances

Ugly duckling stage – 'goofy' spaced teeth (mixed dentition) with teeth appearing to be too large for the face

Wafer – plastic occlusal guide used at osteotomy operations

Wafer impressions – impressions taken to make a wafer

Wax – material used to record the relationship between the upper and lower teeth; also to protect the soft tissues from being rubbed by a fixed appliance

Wisdom teeth – third molars

Work models – models on which appliances are made; not kept as study models

X-rays – needed to produce radiographs

Z spring – spring used on removable appliances to procline incisors

Index

Basic Guide to Orthodontic Dental Nursing, Second Edition. Fiona Grist.
© 2020 John Wiley & Sons Ltd. Published 2020 by John Wiley & Sons Ltd.